D1356216

The Mitchell Beazley Pocket Guide to Nutrition and Calories

Arnold E. Bender

Mitchell Beazley

METRIC EQUIVALENTS AND ABBREVIATIONS

Metric equivalents are approximate throughout (for example, 1oz = 28.4g; this has been rounded up to 30g throughout)

Approximate metric equivalents

1oz = 30g (= 1fl.oz)	6oz = 170g
2oz = 60g	7oz = 200g
4oz = 110g	8oz = 230g
5oz = 140g	1lb = 450g

1 litre = 1¾ pints
1 pint (20fl.oz) = 600ml (6dl)
¼ pint (5fl.oz) = 140ml (1½dl)

N.B. μg = micrograms
mg = milligrams
1,000 calories = kilocalorie (kcal) or Calorie
1,000 joules = kilojoule (kJ)
1,000,000 joules = megajoule (MJ)
1 calorie = 4.2 joules

Edited and designed by
Mitchell Beazley International Limited,
Artists House, 14-15 Manette Street, London W1V 5LB

ISBN 0 85533 676 5

Photoset by MS Filmsetting Limited, Frome,
Somerset, England
Printed and bound in Hong Kong by
Mandarin Offset International Ltd.

1 2 3 4 5 6 7 8 9 10

Editor	David Townsend Jones
Art Editor	Ruth Levy
Production	Androulla Pavlou

Contents

List of tables

Foreword

The science of nutrition is steadily developing, and there is a corresponding increase in the public demand for up-to-date guidance and information. Since the first edition of the *Pocket Guide to Calories and Nutrition* was written there has been a much clearer consensus among scientists on several aspects of nutrition—the need to reduce the consumption of saturated fats, sugar and salt, for instance, and the importance of increasing the consumption of foods that supply dietary fibre.

Similarly the earlier method of assessing overweight according to the size of the body frame—which always encouraged a little cheating anyway—has been replaced by a broader range of acceptable weights. Recent evidence has shown that body weights a little above average are not a health hazard, and it is now accepted that there is a perfectly natural and normal variation between individuals.

This new edition fully reflects these and other significant changes of opinion related to advances in research worldwide, and has been comprehensively revised and updated throughout.

I would like to thank Tony Nash (Dr Nash since the first edition appeared), who initially produced the FOOD COMPOSITION AND CALORIE TABLES on a computer. I would also wish to acknowledge the lasting contributions of Corine Plough and Susannah Read, the editors of the original book, much of whose work is carried forward to this revised edition.

Arnold Bender

Good food – good health

WHAT IS A GOOD DIET?

Different people eat quite different kinds of food—fish and chips, frogs' legs, maize and beans, cassava and peanuts —and all keep quite fit. So what is really meant by a good diet? It is diet that supplies all that is necessary for growth and repair of the body tissues, the energy needed for daily activities, and all the materials needed to enable the body to work properly.

HOW THE BODY UTILIZES FOOD

Foods can be divided into those for: Growth or construction; Energy or fuel; and Function. (And since some foods we eat have little nutritional value we can add a fourth category: foods for fun.)

Growth and construction

A baby born weighing about 6½ lb (3 kg) might after twenty years or so weigh about 130 lb (60 kg). This is a result of diet. Moreover, there is a continuous process of replacing worn-out tissue, even in young people. The materials needed for such construction and repair are *mineral salts* and *proteins*.

Mineral salts, especially calcium and phosphate, together with smaller amounts of other minerals such as magnesium and fluoride, are needed to construct the framework of the body, the skeleton. Calcium cannot be absorbed from the diet into the bloodstream unless vitamin D is present, and this vitamin also helps the deposition of calcium to form bones. Muscles, vital organs, skin and the blood, which carries nutrients around the body, are all made of protein, and since we cannot synthesize protein we have to eat it instead.

Energy and fuel

To explain what nutrition and body function are all about, the body can be likened to a motor-car. The structure— the bodywork and engine—is made largely of protein and minerals, and fuel is needed to supply the energy to make it go. This comes mainly from *carbohydrate* and *fat*. Carbohydrate is the principal fuel for the body; this is its only function. A small proportion of fats is used in tissue structure, but by far the greater part is used for fuel. Additionally, any protein that is not needed for construction can be burned to supply energy.

If you take on board a motor-car more petrol than is

needed it has to be stored in cans in the boot. If you eat more energy foods than the body needs, the excess has to be stored as fat in various parts of the body (not excluding the boot!).

On the other hand, if you fail to take in enough fuel you will gradually use up all the reserves and empty the tank. The body has the additional property of being able to burn up some of its own structural tissues, the muscle proteins, rather as if the motor-car were fitted with wooden seats that could be burned for fuel in an emergency. When all the stored fuel is used and the tanks are empty, and all the disposable tissues have been used up for fuel, then the motor-car cannot go—the body cannot continue to function.

Fortunately most people have a built-in fuel-filling system: they feel hungry when fuel is needed and rarely allow the tank to empty. On the contrary, they are more likely to take too much in and the reserves may grow dangerously large.

Function

Continuing the motor-car analogy, fuel and engine alone are not enough. They cannot work without sparking plugs— the body cannot function without *vitamins*. These are neither materials of construction nor fuel but are needed in very small amounts to permit proper functioning of the body. Some vitamins require the joint function of mineral salts, so these may be considered both structural and functional.

Finally, the importance of *dietary fibre,* or roughage, should also be mentioned. This is a particular type of indigestible carbohydrate material without which the intestine cannot function properly.

7

The essential nutrients

PROTEINS

Proteins are found in foods as diverse as milk, peas, liver, eggs, bread, potatoes and fish. In fact, since proteins are the basis of all living tissues, everything that is grown, plant and animal, contains some protein unless the food has been extracted from its original source. For example, when olive oil is pressed from the olive or sugar extracted from the cane, what is obtained is a pure fat and a pure carbohydrate, although the original olive and the sugar cane did contain some protein. So even cabbage and rhubarb—90 percent water—contain a little protein (2-3 percent), whereas wheat, maize and rice contain about 10 percent, and meat and fish are called rich sources because they contain 20 percent protein.

To put these figures into perspective, a good diet should contain 5-10 percent protein, although most of us prefer to eat a diet of 10-12 percent protein, which is the approximate norm.

You may wonder how proteins from such diverse sources can be used to make human flesh, blood, liver and lungs. The answer is that all proteins are made of 20 basic units, the amino acids, linked together in a variety of combinations. During the process of digestion the proteins are broken down into their constituent amino acids, absorbed into the bloodstream and travel around the body to the places where they are needed. Here they are rebuilt into the particular proteins needed for kidneys, heart, glands and all the other tissues.

So any protein can be used to make human protein. Some, however, must be more useful than others. For example, would it not be more efficient if we were all cannibals so that the protein we ate was the same composition as the protein in the body? Only to a limited extent. Firstly, in the continuous process of breakdown and repair that goes on, tissues like heart and intestine are being broken down and replaced much faster than the muscles and very much faster than the skin and bones, so to eat representative samples of human tissue would not be all that practical. Secondly, it is only when we are eating the bare minimum amount of protein—about 1½ oz (45 g) a day—that we need worry whether the proportions of amino acids in the protein closely resemble those of the body. In the industrialized world we eat two or three times as much protein as this, so even if the amino acid make-up differs considerably from our requirements, quantity

makes up for quality. The body simply selects those amino acids it needs from those that are eaten, and the rest are burned off to provide energy.

CARBOHYDRATES

These are the starchy foods and sugars that make up the greater part of our cereals, pastas, cakes and biscuits. In round figures our diet is about 50 percent carbohydrate, 40 percent fat and 10 percent protein. About one-third of the carbohydrate is sugar—half of this is taken in cups of tea and coffee, and the rest in manufactured and cooked foods.

Bread, the commonest food in many countries, consists of 50 percent carbohydrate, 10 percent protein and 2 percent fat, the rest being water. Bread is often called a starchy food, but from the point of view of protein we could live on bread alone.

Sugar, on the other hand, contains nothing but carbohydrate—it is, in fact, a very pure chemical substance. So when we make flour confectionery by mixing flour (at 10 percent protein) with sugar (zero protein) and fat (also zero protein) we are diluting a good food to a point where it sometimes contributes little to the diet other than energy, with only traces of minerals, vitamins and protein. These must be considered as fun foods rather than as sources of any particular nutrients.

FATS

Fats are fairly obvious as butter, margarine, salad oil and cooking fat, but many other foods also contain fat. Bread has already been mentioned as containing about 2 percent fat; fancy breads can contain more than that, and the level can go as high as 30 percent in some crackers. Then there are milk and cheese, fatty meats and fatty fish. Even in very lean meat there is as much as 10 percent fat between the muscle fibres. Consequently many foods that are not themselves fats do contain quite a lot of fat.

A small amount of fat is essential in the diet—about 10 percent, failing which certain vitamins, such as vitamins A and D, cannot be absorbed into the bloodstream from the digestive tract. In Western communities about 40 percent of the energy we consume is fat. As discussed later, this is thought to be too much for good health. Certainly fat helps the food go down—just imagine trying to swallow dry bread in any quantity—and in many foods the greater part of the flavour is in the fatty part. A further point is that fats are a more concentrated form of energy than carbohydrates and proteins, so that if a diet is very low in fat it will have to be bulkier and will often be too bulky for comfort.

VITAMINS

There are 13 vitamins of known importance to man (Table 1). All are essential to life, but eight are of special

1 Nutritionally important vitamins

Number	Name	
A	Retinol (in animal foods)	
	Carotene (in plant foods)	
B_1	Thiamin	
B_2	Riboflavin	
—	Niacin or nicotinic acid	B-complex
—	Folic acid or Folacin	group
B_6	Pyridoxine	
C	Ascorbic acid	
D	Cholecalciferol	

Less important vitamins

E	Tocopherol
K	Menaphthone
—	Pantothenic acid
B_{12}	Cyanocobalamin
H	Biotin

nutritional importance, since they are in short supply in some communities and some individuals. Deficiencies of the other vitamins are caused not so much through a dietary shortage but because the subject suffers from some disease or is unable to absorb the vitamins from the food.

The nutritionally important vitamins

Vitamin A is needed for growth and to keep the cells that line the various passages of the body in their normal moist condition. Although well-fed people have about two years' supply of the vitamin in their livers, in many developing countries, especially in the southeast Pacific and Middle East, there is a widespread shortage which results in cells becoming dry and hard. If this happens in the eye it damages the cornea and eventually leads to blindness. Another function of vitamin A is to enable us to see in dim light; when the supply is inadequate night-blindness results. It is not, however, involved in vision in full light.

Vitamin A is found in animal foods as retinol, the form used in our bodies. In plant foods it exists in the form of carotene, which is converted into retinol in the walls of the intestine. It is plentiful in a wide variety of foods, including milk, butter, yellow and orange fruit, green vegetables, and particularly in liver and carrots. One carrot weighing 2oz (60g) can contain a 3-day supply of carotene.

B vitamins can be considered together since some have parallel functions and also often occur together in the same foods. For example, meat and cereals contain

vitamin B_1, niacin and some vitamin B_2, and it is present in large amounts in liver and in milk.

So far as function is concerned, vitamins B_1, B_2 and niacin are involved at different stages in the release of energy from foods. The energy is not liberated suddenly, just as a motor-car does not function by setting the petrol ablaze, but through a complex 20-stage system with the aid of these three vitamins.

Vitamin B_6 is concerned with reconstituting amino acids derived from food protein into the proteins of the body. Good sources include meat, especially liver, green vegetables and unrefined cereals.

Folic acid is also found in a wide variety of foods, especially liver and many vegetables; problems seldom arise from a shortage of it. A deficiency results in anaemia.

B-vitamin-deficiency diseases are various, and some of them can be fatal. A serious and prolonged shortage of vitamin B_1 results in beriberi. This disease was very common, and still exists in Far Eastern countries. Victims have difficulty in walking because of damage to the nerves, and the heart is affected. It was shown to be a nutritional disease in the Japanese Navy as long ago as 1883, caused by relying on white rice as the main part of the diet. Whole-grain (or brown) rice contains plenty of vitamin B_1, but it is removed during milling to white rice. This also happens when wheat is milled to white flour, but Western countries obtain their vitamin B_1 from so many other foods that beriberi never occurs. Eastern sufferers do not get these other foods, so beriberi is associated with rice-eating communities.

Pellagra results from a serious deficiency of niacin. It was described 250 years ago and literally means, in Italian, rough skin. This is because it looks like a specific type of dermatitis, particularly on the face, neck and arms, which are exposed to light; there is damage also to the digestive system and the brain. It was many years before the precise dietary problem was identified—at one time it was thought to be caused by harmful substances in maize because it is common in maize-eating areas, then by protein shortage, and, in the 1940s, it was thought to be caused by niacin deficiency. In fact all three theories are correct. One of the amino acids that is present in protein, namely tryptophan, is converted into niacin in the body—and maize is relatively short of both.

Vitamin B_2 and B_6 deficiency may cause cracking of the skin at the corners of the mouth, and soreness of the lips and tongue.

Vitamin C or, rather, scurvy caused by a shortage of vitamin C, has a long history. The vitamin is found in fruit and vegetables, and is largely destroyed by drying, and more slowly during storage.

The people who suffered most from scurvy were sailors who, being away from land for months or even years, had

little fresh food, and sometimes no fruit and vegetables at all. When Vasco da Gama in 1497 sailed around the Cape of Good Hope, 100 out of his crew of 160 died of scurvy. It became known early in the sixteenth century that the juice of certain leaves was a cure, and successful explorers such as Captain Cook stopped at every opportunity to take on board fruit and vegetables. Scurvy was eliminated in the British Navy after 1795 by providing lime juice—hence the name of "limeys" for Britishers.

Although vitamin C is present in all fruit and vegetables the amounts vary enormously, and a lot can be lost in processing and cooking. Black currants, for example, are an extremely rich source containing as much as 200 mg per $3\frac{1}{2}$ oz (100 g), while apples contain only about 5 mg per $3\frac{1}{2}$ oz (100 g). Oranges contain about 50 mg each and leafy vegetables contain 30 to 100 mg per $3\frac{1}{2}$ oz (100 g).

Figures given for vitamin C in foods are very approximate because it is so readily lost. First, we find that the amount originally present in the fresh food can vary a great deal depending on the variety of plant, soil, climate, fertilizer and growing conditions; the fruit on the sunny side of the tree may contain more vitamin C than the rest. Next, there is a steady loss once the crop has been harvested because of self-destruction by an enzyme present in the fruit or vegetable. In the living plant this is kept separate, but when the leaf begins to wilt after cropping or the fruit is slightly bruised, especially in mechanical harvesting and transport, the enzyme comes into contact with the vitamin and it is steadily destroyed.

The next loss takes place during cooking when the greater part can be washed out into the water, the amount depending, of course, on how finely the food is chopped. There is 80 or 90 percent loss from chopped cabbage, but only 20 or 30 percent loss from whole potatoes. Much of this can be recovered from the water, so it is sound practice to use the water for gravies.

The final loss takes place because of oxidation by air when the food is kept hot before eating. Mashed potato, for example, can lose half its remaining vitamin C if kept hot for 20 minutes.

Despite this enormous loss, there is no great likelihood of scurvy in most countries, since half an orange will provide nearly all the vitamin C needed for a day. Most people eat some vegetables, however badly they may be cooked, and fruit, and there is even a little in milk and in jam. Scurvy is the result of severe deficiency; the effects of long-term very slight shortages are unclear.

Vitamin D has the unique distinction of being a nutrient that can be synthesized in the skin under the influence of sunlight. We do not know how much is made under the skin: it obviously depends on how much sunlight reaches how much skin, so we cannot say exactly how much ought to be consumed. It is needed for both absorption of calcium

from the diet into the bloodstream and for the deposition of calcium on the bones.

Therefore a deficiency in growing children, who need to form new bone, and adolescents who are undergoing a growth spurt, can cause rickets. A deficiency is also possible in adults, not from lack of new bone growth but through loss of calcium from existing bones. In adults it is termed osteomalacia and is found in women on a poor diet, sheltered from sunlight by living largely indoors and with repeated pregnancies that call for extra calcium for the growing infant. Such deficiencies in pregnant women are rare in the industrialized world but are common in some developing countries. Probably the greater problem in industrialized countries is that of elderly housebound people, who are consequently without the benefit of sunshine and who, at the same time, eat a diet restricted in variety and particularly lacking in ready-made vitamin D. Problems also occur in the UK in some young children because of lack of the vitamin in their diet, and also, for reasons not yet understood, among adolescent Asian children.

Not many foods contain vitamin D. Fatty fish are a good source, there is some in eggs and butter, and it is added to margarine.

Vitamin B₆ (pyridoxine) in large doses may help to alleviate premenstrual syndrome (PMS). The RDA (see page 20) is only about 2 mg (using the US RDA figure), while the dose used for PMS is 50-100 mg a day for several months. Such large doses cannot simply be correcting a vitamin deficiency but must be functioning, if at all, like a medical drug. The value of B_6 in PMS is therefore by no means certain and it is still under trial.

Folacin is particularly necessary during pregnancy to supply the rapidly growing fetus, and is prescribed by some doctors. There is considerable research into the possibility that a shortage of folic acid in the very first few weeks of pregnancy may be the cause of spina bifida (neural tube defect) in newborn babies. The problem here is that the effects of a shortage occur so early in pregnancy that the vitamin is needed *before* pregnancy occurs.

The less important vitamins

Many people around the world suffer deficiencies of the vitamins discussed above, while deficiencies of the other vitamins are very rare.

For example, nobody, even in the developing countries, has ever been shown to suffer from a shortage of vitamin E. A deficiency can be created in the laboratory on controlled diets, or can occur after surgery or in diseases that prevent absorption of the vitamin, but it seems that all diets, however poor, contain enough.

Another vitamin that almost never seems to be in short supply is vitamin H, or biotin. We do know that it can

become linked to raw egg white and pass straight through the intestine without being absorbed, but it seems you would have to eat an extraordinary diet to create a deficiency, as illustrated by the first and almost only case, which was reported from the United States in 1943. This was an egg farmer who ate six dozen raw eggs a week washed down with a daily dose of 4 quarts (4.5 litres) of red wine (his wife and children left him). He developed a type of dermatitis and finished up in hospital. Since there are many types of dermatitis he was treated with one substance after another until finally he responded to vitamin H. Such eccentrics often provide as much scientific data as carefully planned laboratory experiments.

A dietary shortage of vitamin B_{12} is also very rare; however, some people are unable to absorb it and this is the cause of pernicious anaemia.

MINERAL SALTS

A very large number of mineral salts is needed, but only a few are likely to be undersupplied: these are iron, calcium, iodine, fluorine and zinc.

The nutritionally important minerals

Iron is part of the red colouring material of the blood and when it is in short supply iron-deficiency anaemia results. Mild anaemia is very common, particularly among women, since the loss of blood in menstruation means a loss of iron from the body. It is so common that anaemia is often regarded as the main nutritional deficiency in well-fed countries, but there are recent medical suggestions that mild anaemia is not a problem but just a normal variation between people. It is only when the blood haemoglobin falls well below normal levels that the anaemia becomes severe enough to be regarded as ill health.

Unfortunately iron is not well absorbed from foods: often only 10 percent or less is absorbed. Meat and animal products such as liver and other organ meats are particularly rich in iron that is reasonably well absorbed. Some other foods, such as curry powder, black treacle and cocoa, are relatively rich in iron, but the amount absorbed is very variable and is certainly far less than that absorbed from meat. Vitamin C in amounts of 50-100mg greatly assists the absorption of iron from foods eaten at the same meal.

Calcium itself is usually adequately supplied—the problem is ensuring sufficient vitamin D to help absorb it. We need to consume about one gram of calcium a day, and milk and cheese are the only foods particularly rich in this mineral, unless bread is fortified as in some countries.

Iodine is not obtained in sufficient quantity in certain areas and this shortage results in goitre: the thyroid gland, located in the throat, enlarges and can become big enough to be seen as a large swelling. The iodine content

of plant and animal foods depends on how much there is in the soil, and there is not much in limestone areas, so that goitre is a local problem; it was called "Derbyshire neck" when it was common in that part of England.

The only rich source of iodine in the diet is fish.

Fluorine is a mineral salt, the importance of which lies in protecting teeth from decay. It is always present in bones, teeth and skin, and therefore is a dietary essential, like many other minerals. It has been shown in many parts of the world that where the drinking water has about one part of fluorine per million parts of water dental decay is much less than in areas where there are only traces. That is why it is added to water in some places.

Zinc provides an example of how recent research has revealed properties of nutrients not previously suspected. It was as late as 1960 that zinc deficiency was shown to be a problem in some parts of the world. A deficiency has adverse effects on fertility and delays sexual development in young men. There are traces of zinc in most foods, and good sources include meat and meat by-products, and shellfish.

The less important minerals

Other minerals are rarely, if ever, in short supply: for example, phosphate, sulphate, chloride, sodium, potassium and magnesium are all needed but are plentiful in almost every diet. Although phosphate has often been used as a general "tonic", there is never any likelihood of a shortage and, in fact, UK food regulations prevent manufacturers making any claims for its presence in their products. It is added as a processing aid to meat products such as poultry and sausages because it holds water and keeps them juicy and soft. Magnesium is found in small but adequate amounts in many foods; bran, cocoa and some nuts are rich sources.

For all nutrients, it is true that we are unsure of the effects of long-term very slight deficiencies. Mild shortages may give rise to vague symptoms that are more than difficult to diagnose.

So how can we make sure that we are getting an adequate amount of all the nutrients described above, and what quantity of which foods will supply it? These questions, together with guidelines for a sensible diet, will be dealt with in WHAT SHOULD WE EAT, pages 20–39.

Measuring energy: calories and joules

The energy taken in as food and the energy spent in living are measured in calories and, nowadays, in joules. Both the calorie and joule are rather small units to work with, so we use a unit of 1,000 calories called a kilocalorie (kcal), or Calorie with a capital "C"; a unit of 1,000 joules called a kilojoule (kJ); and a unit of a million joules called a megajoule (MJ). In practice, "calorie" is often written when strictly it should be "Calorie".

One calorie is approximately 4 joules (to be precise, 4.2), so multiplying Calories (kilocalories) by four gives kilojoules.

The energy of food is converted into work with only about 25 percent efficiency; the rest is wasted as heat. Although this may seem rather inefficient, it is about as efficient as the internal combustion engine and much better than the steam engine.

HOW MUCH FUEL DO WE NEED?

The average adult eats and spends about 2,500 Calories (10,000 kilojoules) per day. The energy content of 1g of starch or sugar or any other carbohydrate is 4 Calories (16 kilojoules); that of 1g of protein is 4 Calories (17 kilojoules). (The difference between 16 and 17 is because of rounding off.) The energy content of 1g of fat or oil is 9 Calories (37 kilojoules). That is why fats are a more concentrated form of fuel and why one would need to eat a much bulkier diet to get the same energy from a carbohydrate diet. A loaf of bread weighing just over 1lb (480g) contains, in round figures, 250g starch, 50g protein and 10g fat (plus iron, calcium, and B vitamins). This would supply 1,000 Calories (4,000 kilojoules) from carbohydrate, 200 Calories (850 kilojoules) from protein and 90 Calories (375 kilojoules) from fat—a total of 1,290 Calories (5.25 megajoules) or about half the average daily need of energy.

Table 2 lists a variety of daily, recreational and maximum-effort activities, and shows the energy expenditure per minute of a 154-lb (70-kg) adult on each. Needless to say, cycling and playing games require more energy than walking slowly. If you want to burn up a lot of energy you don't have to ski uphill or walk in loose snow: try running upstairs, which will use up about 20 Calories (80 kilojoules) per minute.

Table 3 is a daily balance sheet of energy input and expenditure for an office worker and for someone em-

ployed in heavy manual work. The table gives Calorie expenditure per minute for each of the office worker's activities and also the total time spent in each activity, so that total daily energy output may be arrived at. As the table shows, even at complete rest he spends 1.1 Calories (4.4 kilojoules) per minute keeping body and soul together, and standing puts up the cost to about 2 Calories

2 Energy expenditure in Calories per minute for a 154-lb (70-kg) adult

Daily activities	Calories per minute
Washing and dressing	2.6–3.0
Walking slowly	2.9
Walking quickly	5.2
Sitting	1.5
Sitting and writing	2.0
Driving car	2.8
Driving motorcycle	3.4
Sweeping floor	1.7
Ironing	4.2
Polishing floor	4.8
Recreation	
Cycling slowly	4.5
Cycling quickly	11.1
Digging	8.6
Playing tennis	7.1
Playing football	8.9
Cricket (fielding)	3.9
Cricket (bowling)	5.2
Cricket (batting)	6.0
Maximum efforts	
Planing hardwood	9
Shovelling earth	10
Sculling at 106yd (97m)/min	11
Swimming at 60yd (55m)/min	14
Climbing with load	13
Skiing uphill	19
Walking in loose snow	20

17

3 Daily energy balance sheet of an office worker Weight 145lb (66kg), height 5ft 6in (168cm)

	Time	Cal/min	Cal*	MJ
Sleep	8hrs	1.1	530	2.2
Off work				
Light sedentary activity	4hrs	1.48	360	1.5
Washing and dressing	½hr	3.0	90	0.4
Light domestic work	1 hr	3.0	180	0.8
Walking	1 hr	6.6	400	1.7
Gardening	25mins	4.8	120	0.5
Standing	20mins	1.56	30	0.1
At work				
Sitting activities	3hrs 10mins	1.65	320	1.3
Standing activities	3hrs 40mins	1.9	420	1.8
Walking	12mins	6.6	80	0.3
TOTALS				
Sleeping			530	2.2
Total working			820	3.4
Total off work			1180	4.9
Total			**2530**	**10.6**
Basal metabolic rate			1680	7.0
Energy intake calculated from diet			2620	11.0

Daily energy balance sheet of a manual worker Weight 145lb (66kg), height 5ft 6in (168cm)

	Cal	MJ
Sleeping	530	2.2
Work	1700	7.1
Remainder	1560	6.5
Total	**3790**	**15.8**
Basal metabolic rate	1680	7.0
Energy intake calculated from diet	3990	16.7

*Total Calories per day (mean of 7 days' measurements)

4 A representative day's diet

Food	Quantity	Energy		Protein
		Cal	MJ	g
Milk	14fl.oz (420ml)	350	1.5	18
Cheese	½oz (15g)	60	0.2	4
Bread & cereals	9oz (270g)	740	3.0	19
Meats	6oz (170g)	420	1.8	21
Fats	1½oz (45g)	370	1.5	0
Sugar & preserves	2½oz (75g)	280	1.2	0
Vegetables	12oz (340g)	180	0.8	7
Fruit	5oz (140g)	60	0.3	1
Totals		**2400**	**10.1**	**66**

(8 kilojoules). (Of course, all the figures given are only averages; some people are more efficient and more economical in their movements, while others are awkward and waste a lot of effort.)

The foods shown in Table 4 would be a representative day's meals, providing about 70g protein and 2,500 Calories (10.5 megajoules).

If your body weight is not changing then you must be taking in the same amount of fuel in the form of food as you are spending in activity (resting metabolism, daily work and recreation). If you are gaining weight you must be taking in more than you are spending; if you take in less you will lose weight. Later on the problems of obesity and dieting are discussed in OBESITY AND SLIMMING (pages 53-61), but it is a fact of life that anyone gaining weight is eating more than he or she is using.

What should we eat?

HOW MUCH OF EACH NUTRIENT?

We eat food, not nutrients, but we need to know how much of each nutrient we require so that we can find how much of which foods we should eat. It is possible to get a good diet—which means to obtain all the essential nutrients—from diets as different as those based on meat and two vegetables, rice and fish, or caterpillars and maize (adequately supplemented with smaller amounts of other foods), since we can get the nutrients we need from very different sources. There is no such thing as a perfect diet, but there are very many good diets adapted to individual likes and dislikes.

It is very difficult, and in the present state of knowledge impossible, to find out exactly what each individual needs—we differ so much from one another. The best that we can do, by examining diets eaten by people who appear to be perfectly well and by experimenting on a limited number of people, is to arrive at figures for the *average* nutritional requirements. It is then possible by adding a safety margin to arrive at an amount that will be enough for everyone—those with low, average and above average needs. If we eat a little of everything, all our needs for the various nutrients are most likely to be met.

WHAT IS RDA?

RDA (or RDI) stands for Recommended Daily Allowances or Amounts (or Intakes). They are the amounts of each nutrient that would satisfy the daily needs of everyone, including those whose needs are above average. They are calculated by measuring in the laboratory the needs of volunteers and taking an average, then adding an extra 20 percent, which is enough for everyone.

RDA's apply only to population groups. They do *not* apply to individuals; one might perhaps need 20 percent less than average, which is 40 percent less than the RDA.

They are used for planning and procuring food supplies for population groups, interpreting food-composition records, establishing standards for public assistance programmes, developing nutrition education programmes, and establishing guidelines for nutritional labelling of foods.

Nutrient requirements, and therefore recommended intakes, differ with sex, age, weight and activity. The extra 20 percent that is added to the average measured requirements does not apply to energy—otherwise people would

presumably get fatter—but to vitamins, minerals and proteins. In any case, people vary enormously in their individual energy expenditure and therefore in their energy needs, and unless they are gaining or losing weight, appetite acts as a mechanism to ensure that their energy intake satisfies their needs.

Although RDA's are calculated on a daily basis, there is no need to worry about getting our nutrients every single day, because our bodies carry a reasonably good reserve of everything we need nutritionally. But there is neither any harm nor, indeed, any benefit to be gained in taking more than the RDA of nutrients.

In fact, those with average needs would get more than their requirements if their diet simply supplied the RDA; even a single carrot, for example, will supply far more than the RDA of vitamin A. However, while there is no harm in consuming more nutrients than we need from food, it is possible to consume excessive and possibly harmful amounts from an overdosage of vitamin preparations.

Measurements of human requirements for nutrients are difficult and complicated. They are made on a sample of only a few people, so the figures cannot be totally accurate. They depend to some extent on the opinions of the particular committee concerned, and there are some variations between tables published in different countries.

Table 5 shows the UK figures, last revised in 1979. Figures are given for men and women at different ages and levels of activity, but in fact apparently similar people differ widely in their needs. Most infants on average eat and need far less than their parents, which is hardly surprising; but there are some who eat and need as much as adults.

In some countries figures are published only for the physiological *need* for protein—6-7 percent of the diet. The UK table rounds this up to 10 percent, since less would be unpalatable; so the table shows that a very active man takes more protein (90g) than a sedentary man (68g). The table assumes that a diet providing enough of the six vitamins for which good information is available will also supply enough B_6 and folic acid, for which there is less information.

WHICH FOODS SUPPLY THE NUTRIENTS?

A look around the supermarket shelves shows what an enormous number of foods are available to us. Except for sugar and starch, which are carbohydrates only, and fats, most foods supply several nutrients. Some foods, however, are richer sources of protein or vitamins or minerals than others.

Energy

Energy is never a problem: almost everyone eats enough to satisfy their appetite and thus satisfy their needs for

5 Recommended Daily Amounts of energy and nutrients for the UK

Age range	Occupational category	Bodyweight		Energy	
		lb	kg	cal	MJ
Boys and girls					
0 up to 1 year		16	7.3	800	3.3
1 up to 2 years		25	11.4	1200	5.0
2 up to 3 years		30	13.5	1400	5.9
3 up to 5 years		36	16.5	1600	6.7
5 up to 7 years		45	20.5	1800	7.5
7 up to 9 years		55	25.1	2100	8.8
Boys					
9 up to 12 years		70	31.9	2500	10.5
12 up to 15 years		100	45.5	2800	11.7
15 up to 18 years		135	61.0	3000	12.6
Girls					
9 up to 12 years		73	33.0	2300	9.6
12 up to 15 years		107	48.6	2300	9.6
15 up to 18 years		124	56.1	2300	9.6
Men					
18 up to 35 years	Sedentary	144	65	2700	11.3
	Moderately active			3000	12.6
	Very active			3600	15.1
35 up to 65 years	Sedentary	144	65	2600	10.9
	Moderately active			2900	12.1
	Very active			3600	15.1
65 up to 75 years	Assuming a sedentary life	139	63	2350	9.8
75 and over		139	63	2100	8.8
Women					
18 up to 55 years	Most occupations	122	55	2200	9.2
	Very active			2500	10.5
55 up to 75 years	Assuming a sedentary life	117	53	2050	8.6
75 and over		117	53	1900	8.0
Pregnancy, 2nd and 3rd trimester				2400	10.0
Lactation				2700	11.3

energy. On the contrary, the problem is that some people eat too much.

Protein

Nor does protein present a problem, because if we eat enough food to satisfy our energy needs we will automati-

* Vitamin B_1 = Thiamin
† Vitamin B_2 = Riboflavin
‡ Vitamin C = Ascorbic Acid

Protein	*B_1	†B_2	Niacin	‡C	A	D	Calcium	Iron
g	mg	mg	mg	mg	µg	µg	mg	mg
20	0.3	0.4	5	15	450	10	600	6
30	0.5	0.6	7	20	300	10	500	7
35	0.6	0.7	8	20	300	10	500	7
40	0.6	0.8	9	20	300	10	500	8
45	0.7	0.9	10	20	300	2.5	500	8
53	0.8	1.0	11	20	400	2.5	500	10
63	1.0	1.2	14	25	575	2.5	700	13
70	1.1	1.4	16	25	725	2.5	700	14
75	1.2	1.7	19	30	750	2.5	600	15
58	0.9	1.2	13	25	575	2.5	700	13
58	0.9	1.4	16	25	725	2.5	700	14
58	0.9	1.4	16	30	750	2.5	600	15
68	1.1	1.7	18	30	750	2.5	500	10
75	1.2	1.7	18	30	750	2.5	500	10
90	1.4	1.7	18	30	750	2.5	500	10
65	1.0	1.7	18	30	750	2.5	500	10
73	1.2	1.7	18	30	750	2.5	500	10
90	1.4	1.7	18	30	750	2.5	500	10
59	0.9	1.7	18	30	750	2.5	500	10
53	0.8	1.7	18	30	750	2.5	500	10
55	0.9	1.3	15	30	750	2.5	500	12
63	1.0	1.3	15	30	750	2.5	500	12
51	0.8	1.3	15	30	750	2.5	500	10
48	0.7	1.3	15	30	750	2.5	500	10
60	1.0	1.6	18	60	750	10	1200	15
68	1.1	1.8	21	60	1200	10	1200	15

cally get enough protein. The only way we could go short of protein is if we took a substantial part of our energy as empty calories—that is, from foods which have little or no nutritional value: too much sugar, too much fat and too much alcohol. (For more about alcohol see the section on ALCOHOL, pages 40-42.) With the usual amounts of sugar, fat and alcohol that are consumed by the average person we still get at least twice as much protein as we need.

Much protein comes from cereals. Bread, flour and foods made from wheat, together with rice, barley, oats and maize, all contain roughly 10 percent protein. There are especially rich sources of protein such as meat, fish, eggs, milk and cheese; even foods rather low in protein such as vegetables and potatoes contribute to the total intake.

Table 6 shows some sources of protein.

Vitamins

We cannot be so certain that our vitamin intake is adequate, although given the types of food eaten in the Western world it is most unlikely that there would be a shortage severe enough to give rise to deficiency diseases. What is more likely is that we might not get quite enough and be below maximum efficiency and optimum health without realising it. Then when some infection such as influenza comes along or we break a leg it might take longer to recover. This is more than difficult to prove and the only way to make sure that we are getting enough is to eat all the right foods.

The water-soluble vitamins of the B complex and vitamin C, unlike vitamins A and D, are not much stored in the body, so a deficiency can arise within a few weeks. While it is by no means essential to consume these vitamins every day at every meal, it is advisable to consume them fairly regularly. Vitamins A and D, on the other hand, could, if one wanted, be eaten once a week or

6 Sources of protein

Food	Protein:	g/oz*	g/100g†
Dried skimmed milk		10	35
Sunflower seeds		8	28
Peanuts		8	28
Cheese (Cheddar)		7	25
Dried full-cream milk		7	25
Green peas (dry)		7	25
Haricot beans (dry)		7	25
Almonds		6	21
Beef		5	18
Codfish		5	18
Evaporated milk		2	7
Green peas (fresh)		1.6	6
Milk		0.9	3

*grams of protein per oz   †grams of protein per 100g

even less frequently.

Vitamin A The needs of an adult will be satisfied with
about 750 micrograms of this vitamin a day. It is found in
very large amounts in carrots and liver: $3\frac{1}{2}$oz (100g) of
either would keep us going for a week or more. Milk,
butter, egg yolk, cheese, tomatoes, all green vegetables,
and yellow and orange fruit such as apricots, peaches and
melons also supply vitamin A. Countries in which dairy
produce and meat supplies are scarce rely heavily upon
vegetable and fruit sources as an alternative. Any surplus
of vitamin A is stored in the liver, so most people have a
good reserve. For good sources of the vitamin, see Table 7
below.

B vitamins The RDA of an adult for vitamin B_1 is about
1mg. We can get about a third of this from 2oz (60g) of
meat, bacon or heart, $1\frac{1}{2}$oz (45g) of peanuts or 2oz (60g) of
oatmeal. Cereals are good sources of vitamin B_1. White
bread in many countries is enriched with added vitamin

7 Good sources of vitamin A

Portions supplying one-third of RDA for an adult

Food *(as preformed vitamin A or retinol)*	Portion
Halibut-liver oil	1 drop (50mg)
Cod-liver oil	$\frac{1}{4}$teaspoon (1g)
Liver (sheep and ox)	$\frac{1}{3}$oz (10g)
Liver (calf)	1oz (30g)
Butter (average)	1oz (30g)
Margarine	1oz (30g)
Eggs	2 eggs (100g)
Milk	$\frac{1}{2}$ pint (3dl)
Food *(as carotene)*	
Red palm-oil	$\frac{1}{6}$oz (5g)
Carrots (old)	$\frac{1}{3}$oz (10g)
Carrots (new, tinned)	$\frac{2}{3}$oz (20g)
Spinach	$\frac{2}{3}$oz (20g)
Apricots (dried)	2oz (60g)
Watercress	$\frac{2}{3}$oz (20g)
Broccoli	$3\frac{1}{2}$oz (100g)
Tomatoes	2oz–1lb (60–450g)
Maize	$2\frac{1}{4}$lb (1kg)
Peppers (red)	$3\frac{1}{2}$oz (100g)
Peppers (green)	1lb (450g)
Cabbage	10oz (300g)

B_1 so that 6oz (180g) of this, or 5oz (150g) of wholemeal bread will supply one-third of the daily B_1.

Vitamin B_2 is found in large supply in milk and liver— $\frac{2}{3}$ pint (4dl) of milk or $\frac{3}{4}$oz (20g) of liver will provide a third of the daily need, and there is some to be found also in tea and eggs.

Niacin is needed in a quantity of about 18mg a day. It is found in peanuts, bread, meat and coffee.

Yeast and yeast extract are very rich in vitamins B_1, B_2 and niacin. About $\frac{1}{2}$oz (15g) of brewer's yeast will supply one-third of the RDA.

Good sources of folic acid include liver, spinach and fish, and it is also found in green vegetables, wholemeal bread and eggs. Vitamin B_6 is widely distributed, but good sources include meat, especially liver, green vegetables and wholemeal bread.

Vitamin C The recommended daily intake of vitamin C is about 30-45mg. It is commonly found in all fruit and vegetables, and Table 11 (page 28) shows that some are so rich in it that we could get all we need for a day from 4-5oz (110-140g) of grapefruit or orange, or as little as 1oz (30g) of peppers, black currants or parsley. Potatoes are unusual because while they are not a rich source of vitamin C they

8 Good sources of niacin

Portions supplying one-third of RDA for an adult (6mg)

Food	Portion
Peanuts and peanut butter	1¾oz (50g)
Bread (wholemeal)	7oz (200g)
Yeast (baker's)	⅔oz (20g)
Yeast (brewer's)	½oz (15g)
Rice (white)	20oz (600g)
Rice (parboiled)	10oz (300g)
Soya flour	10oz (300g)
Meats	5oz (140g)
Mushrooms (dried)	3oz (90g)
Liver	2oz (60g)
Barley (pearled)	8oz (230g)
Coffee	⅓oz (10g)
Beer, mild	2 pints (1 liter)
Pulses	10oz (300g)
Sunflower seed	3½oz (100g)
Yeast extract	⅓oz (10g)
Meat extract	½oz (15g)

9 Good sources of vitamin B₁

Portions supplying one-third of RDA for an adult (about 0.3mg)

Food	Portion
Heart (ox)	2oz (60g)
Bacon (lean)	2oz (60g)
Pork (lean)	1¾oz (50g)
Pork (fat)	2½oz (75g)
Cod's roe	¾oz (20g)
Liver and kidney	4oz (110g)
Pulses	1½oz (45g)
Peanuts	1½oz (45g)
Potatoes	10oz (300g)
Oatmeal	2oz (60g)
Flour (wholemeal)	3oz (90g)
Flour (white, enriched)	4oz (110g)
Soya flour	½oz (15g)
Brazil nuts	1oz (30g)
Yeast (baker's)	½oz (15g)
Yeast (brewer's)	⅒oz (3g)
Bread (wholemeal)	5oz (140g)
Bread (white, enriched)	6oz (180g)
Bread (wheatgerm)	¾oz (20g)

10 Good sources of vitamin B₂

Portions supplying one-third of RDA for an adult (about 0.5mg)

Food	Portion
Milk (cow's)	⅔ pint (4dl)
Hard cheese	3½oz (100g)
Liver	¾oz (20g)
Kidney	1oz (30g)
Tea leaves	2oz (60g)
Skimmed milk powder	1oz (30g)
Egg	5oz (140g)
Almonds	2½oz (75g)
Yeast (baker's)	1oz (30g)
Yeast (brewer's)	½oz (15g)
Soft curd-cheese	6oz (170g)

11 Sources of vitamin C
(Raw, edible portion, unless otherwise stated)

Food	mg/oz (30g)
Apples (eating, raw)	1
Bananas	3
Beansprouts	8
Beetroot (cooked)	2
Black currants (raw)	56
Black currants (cooked or tinned)	40
Breadfruit	6
Cabbage (raw)	18
Cabbage (cooked 5 mins)	6
Cabbage (cooked, kept hot 30 mins)	3
Gooseberries	12
Grapefruit juice (in carton)	12
Grapefruit (whole)	5
Grapefruit (peeled, fresh)	12
Guava	56
Horseradish	34
Kale, broccoli, beet, greens, turnip tops	34
Leeks	6
Lemons (whole)	6
Lemons (juice)	12
Lettuce	4
Mango	8
Melon	8
Mustard and cress	20
Okra	7
Oranges (whole)	10
Oranges (peeled)	15
Oranges (juice in carton)	12
Parsley	44
Paw-paw	14
Peas (raw)	7
Peas (fresh, cooked)	4
Peas (tinned, cooked)	3
Peas (dried by modern methods, cooked)	3
Peppers (green or red)	43

mg/100g	Portions supplying 25mg
4	1½lb (700g)—3 large apples
10	9oz (270g)
30	3oz (90g)
6	¾lb (340g)—1 large
200	½oz (15g)—½ tablespoon
140	¾oz (20g)—1 tablespoon
21	4oz (110g)
60	1½oz (45g)—1 cupful
20	5oz (140g)
10	8oz (230g)
40	2oz (60g)
42	2fl.oz (60ml)—wineglassful
17	5oz (140g)—½ small
42	2oz (60g)—8 sections
200	½oz (15g)
120	¾oz (20g)
120	¾oz (20g)
20	4oz (110g)
20	4oz (110g)—1 large
42	2fl.oz (60ml)—wineglassful
14	6oz (170g)—1 large
30	3oz (90g)
30	3oz (90g)
80	1oz (30g)
24	3½oz (100g)
35	2½oz (75g)—½ small orange
50	1½oz (45g)—4-5 sections
42	2fl.oz (60ml)—wineglassful
150	½oz (15g)
50	2oz (60g)
24	3½oz (100g)
15	6oz (170g)
10	8oz (230g)
10	8oz (230g)
150	½oz (15g)

continued on next page

29

Sources of vitamin C

continued from previous page
(Raw, edible portion, unless otherwise stated)

Food	mg/oz (30g)
Pineapple (fresh)	7
Pineapple (juice in carton)	3
Plantain	6
Potatoes (new, cooked)	5
Potatoes (old, after January)	1
Red currants	12
Rosehip syrup	56
Spring onions	7
Sprouts (raw)	28
Sprouts (cooked)	10
Strawberries	17
Swede (cooked)	5
Sweet potato	8
Tomato (raw, cooked or juice)	7
Watercress	18
West Indian cherry	570
Yams (fresh)	3

are eaten by the pound rather than the ounce and so supply a large proportion of the vitamin in the diet of many people. One of the problems, as discussed previously (page 12), is that vitamin C can easily be lost in cooking-water and through numerous other factors, so it pays, in every respect, to be a careful cook.

Vitamin D Very few foods contain vitamin D and there is a possible shortage in children and adolescents who have a special need for bone growth, and in elderly people who are housebound and get little or no vitamin D from sunshine. The recommended intake is about 2·5 micrograms for both adults and children. The richest sources are fatty fish such as sardines, mackerel and pilchards, and it is added to margarine in many countries, to milk in the United States, and is also present in eggs, butter and liver. For good sources, see Table 12 on page 32.

Minerals

Absolute proof that our mineral intake is adequate is impossible, but just as with vitamins, anyone living on a Western diet is most unlikely to suffer from severe mineral-shortage leading to deficiency diseases. Again, the only way to ensure we are getting enough is to eat all

Note: *The vitamin content of foods, and especially vitamin C, varies considerably from one sample to another, and the figures can be used only as a guide.*

mg/100g	Portions supplying 25mg
24	3½oz (100g)—1 slice ½in thick
10	½ pint (3dl)
21	4oz (110g)
18	5oz (140g)—2 med size
4	1½lb (700g)
40	2oz (60g)
200	½fl.oz (15ml)—2 teaspoons
25	3½oz (100g)
100	1oz (30g)—2-3 sprouts
35	2½oz (75g)—5-6 sprouts
60	1½oz (45g)
18	5oz (140g)—large portion
28	3oz (90g)
25	3-4oz (90-110g)—1-2 large tomatoes
60	1½oz (45g)
2000	1 small cherry
10	9oz (270g)

the right foods. However, if the diet is sufficiently varied so that it supplies enough iron, calcium, iodine, fluorine and zinc, it will almost certainly provide enough of all the other minerals needed.

Iron We can get one-third of our daily needs of iron from as little as 1oz (30g) of liver or kidney, or 3½oz (100g) of beef, or from 5oz (140g) of wholemeal bread or 8oz (230g) of enriched white bread. A teaspoon of curry powder, a tablespoon of cocoa or a tablespoon of treacle will also provide a third of the daily needs since they are rich sources, and most vegetables supply small amounts. The recommended daily intake is about 10-15mg. For good sources, see Table 13 on page 33.

Calcium We need about 500mg of calcium a day. Portions of food that supply one-third of this would be 5fl.oz (140ml) fresh milk, between ½oz (15g) and 3½oz (100g) of cheese, depending on the type, and about 7oz (200g) of enriched white bread—there is little calcium in (unenriched) wholemeal bread.

One of the more unusual sources of calcium is the bones of fish. Some kinds, especially canned fish, are eaten with their bones and we could get one-third of our day's needs from as little as ⅓oz (10g) of some dried fish or 2oz (60g) of sardines. For good sources, see Table 14 on page 34.

Iodine and fluorine The main source of iodine is fish, and if fish is eaten once or twice a week there should be no deficiency. It may also be obtained from vegetables, milk and cereals, and it is usually possible to buy salt that has been enriched with iodine.

Fluorine is obtained mainly from drinking water, but there are also small amounts in food, especially fish, and tea. It is added to water in some places, although there appears to be a quite unreasonable opposition to such enrichment by some sections of the public.

Zinc There are traces of zinc in most foods, but good sources are wholemeal bread, hard cheeses, cocoa, meats, meat by-products, and shellfish, especially oysters.

12 Good sources of vitamin D
Portions supplying 1μg

Food	Portion
Cod-liver oil	few drops (0.5g)
Fatty fish:	
Sprats	$\frac{1}{16}$oz (2g)
Herrings and kippers	$\frac{1}{8}$oz (5g)
Mackerel	$\frac{1}{8}$oz (5g)
Salmon (fresh or tinned)	$\frac{1}{4}$oz (7g)
Sardines	$\frac{1}{2}$oz (15g)
Eggs	1 oz (30g)—$\frac{1}{2}$ egg
Egg yolk	$\frac{1}{2}$oz (15g)
Margarine	$\frac{1}{2}$oz (15g)
Butter	5oz (140g)
Liver	3oz (90g)

Amounts supplying 20μg of vitamin D

5 sprats	
2 herring fillets	
2 kipper fillets	
$\frac{1}{2}$oz (15g) eels	
2 teaspoons cod-liver oil	
1 small tin of salmon	
4 eggs	
1 large tin of sardines	
8oz (230g) margarine	

DIETARY FIBRE

There is more to food than fats, proteins and other nutrients. For proper functioning of the intestine we need dietary fibre, or roughage. This is largely a type of carbohydrate material that cannot be digested and so passes along the digestive tract, giving the intestines something to work on.

13 Good sources of iron

Portions supplying one-third of RDA for an adult (4-5mg)

Food	Portion
Curry powder	$\frac{1}{6}$oz (5g)—1 teaspoon
Cocoa powder	1oz (30g)—1 heaped tablespoon
Baked beans	7oz (200g)—1 small tin
Beans and peas (dry)	2$\frac{1}{2}$oz (75g)—half teacup
Lentils (dry)	2oz (60g)
Corned beef	1$\frac{1}{4}$oz (35g)—1 slice
Liver or kidney	1oz (30g)—1 thin slice
Beef (cooked)	3$\frac{1}{2}$oz (100g)
Fish (fried)	12oz (340g)
Sardines	3$\frac{1}{2}$oz (100g)—1 small tin
Oatmeal	3oz (90g)
Cornflakes, etc.	5oz (140g)
Almonds	3$\frac{1}{2}$oz (100g)
Heart	3oz (90g)
Soya flour	2oz (60g)—2 tablespoons
Shellfish	1$\frac{1}{4}$oz (35g)
Treacle	1$\frac{1}{2}$oz (45g)—1 tablespoon
Bread (wholemeal)	5oz (140g)
Bread (white)	8oz (230g)
Wheatgerm	1$\frac{3}{4}$oz (50g)
Green peas	8oz (230g)
Greens (cooked)	12oz (340g)
Greens (raw)	12oz (340g)
Yam and potatoes	12oz (340g)
Flour (white)	7oz (200g)
Flour (wholemeal)	4oz (110g)
Figs and apricots (dry)	3oz (90g)
Prunes (dry)	6oz (170g)
Pasta (dry)	10oz (300g)

14 Good sources of calcium
Portions supply about 200mg

Food	Portion
Milk	⅓ pint (190ml)
Cheese	
Parmesan	½oz (15g)
Cheddar	1oz (30g)
Edam	1oz (30g)
Stilton	2oz (60g)
Whitebait (whole)	⅔oz (20g)
Sprats (whole)	1oz (30g)
Sardines	2oz (60g)
Pilchards (tinned)	3oz (90g)
Soya beans	3oz (90g)
Tripe	5oz (140g)
Molasses	1½oz (45g)
Almonds	3oz (90g)
Kale	3oz (90g)
Broccoli	7oz (200g)
Haricot beans	4oz (110g)
White bread (enriched)	8oz (230g)
White flour (enriched)	5oz (140g)
White flour (unenriched)	3lb (1⅓kg)

RDA for adults is 500mg, for children 600mg.

Fruit contains roughage as pectin, vegetables contain some as cellulose, but the most important and useful source is the bran of cereals, particularly in whole-grain cereals like wholemeal bread. Table 15 (page 36) shows principal sources of dietary fibre.

The value of roughage in the diet in helping to prevent constipation has been known (and ignored) for very many years, but recently a number of diseases growing more common in Western industrialized society have been linked with a shortage of roughage. We are eating much less bread, most of that is white (there is less fibre in white bread than in wholemeal), and the total amount of fibre in the diet is becoming less and less. Many people feel an immediate improvement in preventing constipation by eating bran as breakfast cereal, but other disorders that are not so obvious have been linked to a low-fibre diet. For example, it has been suggested that certain types of cancer of the intestine, varicose veins, heart disease and diabetes are linked with low-fibre diets, but this is not so easy to prove.

It is impossible to say just how much bran anyone should eat. Each person has to find out their own needs. If you are constipated, try taking three or four teaspoons of bran a day, increasing this to perhaps nine or ten teaspoons until the condition is alleviated. Remember that some of the bran breakfast cereals, which many people prefer to ordinary bran, have had sugar and flavour added, so you need about one and a half times as much as you would of ordinary bran.

Apart from bran itself, wholemeal bread is the best source of dietary fibre. Wholemeal bread is made from the whole wheat grain with all its bran: a slice of wholemeal bread is about equivalent to two teaspoons of bran. It is not the same to eat "brown" breads, which are usually partway between white and wholemeal; they may differ considerably in their bran content and will have much less than wholemeal bread.

A good idea would be to eat some wholemeal bread each day, take bran for breakfast and include it in recipes, and eat plenty of fruit and vegetables.

ARE WE PROPERLY FED?

Since the beginning of this century we have learned a great deal about vitamins, mineral salts and proteins, and we have a reasonable idea of how much the average person needs. We also have a very highly developed food industry, well-stocked supermarkets, cookbooks by the thousand and restaurants of all types. Are we all then properly nourished?

The answer is no, on two counts. Firstly, there is no guarantee that everyone is getting all the nutrients he or she needs, and secondly, there has been an enormous increase, in those very countries where these great food improvements have been taking place, in a whole range of diseases that seem to be connected with the diet. They are even called "diseases of affluence". They are due to many different factors, but diet does seem to be involved. They include heart disease, which has been increasing at an alarming rate over the past two generations in all industrialized communities; it seems that the richer people get, the "better" food they eat, but the more they worry about getting richer, the more deaths there are from heart disease. There have been similar increases in diseases of the bowel, including diverticulitis, cancer of the colon, and a group of related diseases. The same goes for obesity, dental decay and diabetes. Certainly some of these are partly inherited, but since it is now too late to change your parents, what can be done?

The rise in these disorders seems to have run parallel to an increased amount of fat in our diets. In many industrialized countries we now take between 40 and 45 percent of our energy from fats, and these are mostly animal fats in meat, milk, butter and cream. We have also

15 Principal sources of dietary fibre

Food	g/3½oz (100g)
Wheat bran	45
Wheat flour (white)	3
Bread (wholemeal)	9
Bread (white)	3
Rice (boiled)	1
Porridge (cooked)	1
All-Bran	27
Cornflakes	3
Muesli	about 7
Shredded Wheat	12
Mustard and cress	4
Parsnips	4
Peas (garden)	5
Peas (processed)	8
Chick peas (cooked)	6
Beans (French, cooked)	3
Plantain (boiled)	6
Spinach (boiled)	6
Corn on the cob (boiled)	5
Apricots (stewed)	9
Blackberries (stewed)	6
Black currants (stewed)	7
Figs (dry)	20
Prunes (stewed)	8
Raisins	7
Raspberries	7
Potatoes	2
Potato crisps	12

been increasing fats in ice cream, cakes and salad dressings. A high level of cholesterol in the blood, which has been shown to be a factor in atherosclerosis, is related to the amount and kind of fat in the diet. Fats, especially saturated fats in animal foods, increase the amount of cholesterol in the blood.

We have also increased our sugar until it amounts to a fifth of the total food-intake (that is an average; some eat far more sugar than this), and we have been eating less and less food that contains any form of dietary fibre.

A SENSIBLE APPROACH

Obviously we cannot go through life selecting and weighing out the foods listed in the tables—it would cause havoc in a restaurant and offend any hostess. How then can we try to make sure that we eat the right foods in sufficient quantity to get all the nutrients we need?

The first point to bear in mind is that if you eat a wide variety of foods there is more chance of your obtaining all the different nutrients. This may sound elementary, because most people eat a varied diet just because they like different food, but there are some people who live on a very monotonous and restricted diet who may well develop shortages of some nutrients.

The second point is to avoid diluting the diet with "empty calories": reduce sugar and sweet foods, reduce fats and oils, and keep alcoholic drinks down to a reasonable level (see ALCOHOL, pages 40-42). There is certainly nothing wrong with an occasional large helping of cake, dessert or fatty foods, or with an occasional drink—unless, of course, you are trying to lose weight (see OBESITY AND SLIMMING, pages 53-61).

DIETARY GOALS

Nutritionists recommend up to six basic dietary modifications that they consider desirable for good health. These are: if you are overweight, lose the excess; eat less fat; eat less sugar; take more dietary fibre; take less salt; and moderate your alcohol intake. Dietary changes such as these cannot do us any harm, and are likely (although, of course, not by any means certain) to reduce the risk of heart disease and bowel complaints, and possibly also of stroke, blood pressure, and other disorders.

How to set about it

You can hardly be expected to change your eating habits overnight. After all, it took a lifetime to acquire them, and you can expect to need some time to change them.

You may find it easier to tackle it in stages: gradually take a little less sugar in your tea and coffee, eat fewer sweets and sweet food, buy leaner meat, have less fat on your bread, change to brown bread, use less salt and salty foods, and eat more fruit and vegetables.

You should be aiming to get by with a little less rather than setting yourself a target of *never* eating *any* of the "less healthy" foods. Even slimmers are "allowed" the occasional half a chocolate éclair or a small glass of wine. "Moderation in all things" should be the rule—even in improving your eating habits.

What it all means

Lose weight The dangers of overweight, recommendations for how to lose it and methods of prevention are discussed in OBESITY AND SLIMMING (pages 53-61). Many illnesses are made more serious by being overweight even if they do not result directly from obesity. A prime requirement for better health, then, is to maintain your correct weight.

Less fat It may never be proved that "too much" fat is a prime cause of many modern diseases, but it is generally accepted that we would all benefit from taking less fat.

But how much is "too much"? The Department of Health Committee on Medical Aspects of Food Policy (COMA) reported in 1984 that the average British consumption of fats was 100g per day (42 percent of the total calorie intake) and recommended that this should be reduced to between 77 and 87g per day (31-35 percent of the total calorie intake).

The reason for this advice is that it has been established that a high intake of fats, particularly of the saturated fats from animal foods, increases the level of cholesterol in the blood. Since high levels of blood cholesterol are considered to be a risk factor in heart disease a reduction in fat-consumption should be beneficial. Saturated fats, the worst offenders, are present in meat and milk, and so in butter and cream.

Some vegetable oils contain polyunsaturates that can reduce the blood cholesterol-level, and it is therefore a good idea to substitute polyunsaturates (as in the special margarines and cooking oils) for saturated fats. But avoid simply adding extra polyunsaturates to your diet—the aim, after all, is to eat altogether less fat.

Less sugar Sugar has been blamed for numerous problems, ranging from obesity and dental decay to diabetes and heart disease. Although none of this is scientifically proved, authorities advise taking less sugar: you should aim to reduce it by half.

The strongest criticism of sugar is that it contains only "empty calories". This means that sugar provides only energy without any nutrients, unlike other foods such as bread, potatoes, fruits and vegetables which supply protein, vitamins and minerals as well as energy.

More dietary fibre Constipation and possibly many other bowel disorders are helped by extra dietary fibre. It comes from whole-grain cereals, for which the chief source is wholemeal bread, and a significant amount is found even in milled cereals and white bread, as well as in all kinds of fruits and vegetables.

Nutritionists recommend a 50-percent increase in dietary fibre. Part of this can be achieved by taking a bran preparation, but some people whose systems cannot tolerate bran may need instead a medicinal form of fibre.

For anyone suffering from constipation there is no actual prescribed "dose" of bran. Each person has to find how much he or she needs. Start with half a dozen teaspoons of bran a day and gradually increase this amount until the problem disappears. You should also eat more potatoes, bread, root crops, fruit and vegetables as sources of fibre to make up for eating less fat and sugar.

Less salt We all take five to ten times more salt than we really need. Although it is still debated whether there is positively any benefit from taking less salt, it seems that it cannot actually cause any harm. Our food already contains enough natural salt to which we add more during cooking and often even more at the table. Moreover, many manufactured foods contain salt. So there is clearly ample scope for reducing our salt intake.

Moderate alcohol Nutritionists seem to keep telling us what is bad for us, so it may be a relief to be told that alcohol—in moderation, of course—is actually beneficial. It helps in promoting healthy blood-flow and to some extent in preventing the formation of blood clots (thrombosis) caused by weakness of the blood platelets.

Excessive alcohol, on the other hand, is harmful because it damages the liver and brain; in the long run it is a killer. Guidelines are provided in Table 16—although (at least some) women may be disappointed to learn that their "ration" is smaller than that of men.

16 Moderate amounts of alcohol

	Alcohol	Spirits		Wine		Beer
	gm	ml	fl.oz	ml	fl.oz	
Men	34	100	3½	340	12	2 pints (1 litre)
Women	23	70	2½	230	8	1¼ pints (700ml)

Excessive amounts

Men	80	240	8½	800	28	4 pints (2 litres)
Women	50	160	5½	500	20	2¾ pints (1½ litres)

WHAT ABOUT CHOLESTEROL?

There is a great deal of confusion between cholesterol in the diet and cholesterol in the blood. A high-fat diet (especially the saturated fats) increases the amount of cholesterol in the blood and so increases the risk of coronary and heart disease. Cholesterol in food, however, has little if any effect on blood levels of cholesterol, and the UK authorities state that they do not make any recommendations about limiting or reducing dietary cholesterol. Certain patients may be put on a low-cholesterol diet, but such changes are not suggested for the general public.

Authorities in the USA advise limiting dietary cholesterol to 300mg a day. The average British intake is 350-450mg, and the UK view is that this amount does not matter. This difference illustrates just how unsure we actually are about the role of cholesterol in the diet.

Alcohol

From the earliest days man discovered how to ferment carbohydrates with yeast and so make alcohol. When we talk about alcohol as a drink we always mean ethyl alcohol, but some people have poisoned themselves by drinking methyl alcohol, also called wood spirit. Around the world there are many different varieties of drinks—even fermented milk such as kumiss and kefir—but most of them fall into one of the three main groups: beer, wines, or spirits.

They differ mainly in their alcoholic content—as any-

17 Nutritional value of alcoholic drinks

	Alcohol (%)	Sugar (%)
Lager	2.6	1.6
Mild beer	2.6	1.6
Stout (bottled)	2.9	4.2
Cider (dry)	3.8	2.6
Cider (sweet)	3.8	4.3
Wine (red/white)	9.0	0.3
Wine (sweet)	10.0	6.0
Port	16.0	12.0
Sherry	16.0	1–7
Spirits	30.0	0
Cherry brandy	19.0	30
Curacao	30.0	30

18 Nutritional value of soft drinks

	Sugar (%)
Colas	10
Grapefruit or orange juice (unsweetened)	8
Grapefruit or orange juice (sweetened)	10
Pineapple juice	13
Lemonade (bottled)	6
Tomato juice	3
Fruit drinks (diluted with 4 parts water)	6

one knows when drinking beer by the pint, wine by the glass and spirits in smaller glasses. Beer, ale and stout are mostly 2-3-percent alcohol together with some carbohydrate (except in beer made specially for diabetics). Wines are mostly 9 to 10-percent alcohol but may contain 8 to 13 percent depending on how much sugar there was in the grapes. The alcohol content, however, cannot go much above 13 percent even when sugar is added to the fruit, because the alcohol kills off the yeast. Sherry and port are fortified by adding brandy and so are about 15-percent alcohol. Spirits such as brandy, whisky and gin are 30-percent alcohol, which is about as strong a solution of alcohol as the mouth can stand. They are made by distilling the alcohol from wine and then diluting it.

In some countries the alcohol content is labelled as

Energy per 3½ fl. oz (100 ml)		Energy per pint (½ litre)	
Cal	kJ	Cal	kJ
25	104	125	520
25	104	140	600
40	160	200	800
35	150	200	870
40	170	240	1000
70	290		
90	400		

Energy per 2 fl. oz (60 ml)	
90	400
70	290
130	550
150	630
190	800

Energy per 3½ fl. oz (100 ml)		Energy per 7 fl. oz (200 ml)	
Cal	kJ	Cal	kJ
40	170	80	340
30	130	60	260
40	170	80	350
50	220	100	440
20	80	40	170
15	70	30	140
20	80	40	170

degrees "proof spirit" instead of by percentage. "Proof spirit" in the UK is 57-percent alcohol by volume and in the USA it is 50 percent. So pure alcohol is 175 degrees proof in the UK and 200 degrees proof in the USA. This is why the same bottle of whisky can be labelled 70 degrees proof (UK) and 84 degrees proof (USA).

"Proof spirit" was a term invented before chemists were as skilled as they are today. It is the strength of alcohol that will ignite when mixed with gunpowder. In the old days, that was when we paid tax; now the chemists are more skilled we pay tax on all alcoholic drinks.

There is no doubt that alcohol is a chemical that is foreign to our bodies, that it is a poison, and that regular, excessive drinking is harmful and can lead to chronic alcoholism. But few people suffer any harm from taking alcoholic drinks in moderation. Social drinking "lifts the spirit, loosens the tongue and removes the inhibitions, so enhancing social intercourse"—and general enjoyment.

Table 17 (pages 40-41) shows several categories of alcoholic drink.

Drinks have very little nutritional value. Spirits provide nothing but energy. Beer does supply a reasonable amount of two of the B vitamins: between 1.5 and 4mg niacin per pint ($\frac{1}{2}$ litre), depending on the strength, which is 10-20 percent of the RDA, and also about 10-20 percent of the RDA of vitamin B_2.

Wines have no more than mere traces of vitamins, but they do contain some iron: a wine glass ($3\frac{1}{2}$ fl. oz or 100 ml) will supply about 1mg of iron, which is 10 percent of the RDA; and the iron in wine appears to be well absorbed. Thus if you drink you would do better to stick to beer or wine—getting some nutrients along with the calories.

You can work out from Table 17 that two glasses of whisky (with or without soda) before a meal, three glasses of wine during it and a glass of liqueur afterwards will give you, in round figures, 650 Calories (2,500 kilojoules)—about as much as a small meal.

There is evidence that alcohol taken in moderation helps blood circulation and strengthens the blood platelets. These are small cells that help the blood to clot when bleeding occurs, but if they break down too easily they can cause blood clots, or thrombosis, in the arteries. So moderate amounts of alcohol can be actually helpful.

The problem is to decide just how much is "moderate". It is well established that, leaving aside the social consequences, too much alcohol can lead to heart disease, can damage the liver and brain, and, long-term, is often fatal.

A recent recommendation came from the committee advising the UK Department of Health. While not saying that alcohol is actually beneficial, the committee reported that a certain amount can be taken with safety. General guidelines on "moderate" amounts of alcohol are provided in Table 16 on page 39.

Fresh or processed food?

BETTER OR WORSE?

Many people who are concerned about their diets will look for fresh rather than processed food. Are they right? The answer is that some fresh foods are better than processed foods, some are worse and others are the same.

Firstly, it must be kept in mind that some losses are intentional, such as when vegetables are trimmed, or fish eviscerated, or foodstuffs such as olive oil or sugar are extracted from the olive or the sugar cane, or when wheat is milled to white flour. The part that is lost is unwanted.

Secondly, cooking is itself a process that causes inevitable losses. Heat always destroys some small part of the nutrients, and severe heat, such as in roasting and baking, causes greater losses. Some part of the water-soluble nutrients, particularly vitamin C in fruit and vegetables, and vitamin B_1 in meat, is washed out into the cooking water, but they are saved, of course, if the cooking juices are consumed.

Thirdly, a lot of our manufactured foods are canned or bottled and come to us ready-cooked. Any losses that may take place in the factory are then *instead* of those that would inevitably take place in our own kitchens, not *additional* to them. By the time the foods reach our plates they probably do not differ much in nutritional content whether they were processed in the factory or cooked at home. So much depends on how fresh the food was to start with, how good the cook is compared with the factory, and whether we really prefer maximum nutritional content to good taste. The very nice taste of roast meat is due largely to damaged protein, but nobody is going to say that roasting should be banned. In any case, the losses are small and anyone who eats meat is not going to suffer from protein shortage.

Then there is the question of what is meant by "fresh foods". They can be garden-fresh, meaning just-harvested, or market-fresh, meaning that a week or more may have passed since they were harvested. Generally the manufacturer starts with garden-fresh food, while the home cook may have to put up with vegetables that are rather stale and tired. Frozen fish is often frozen and even cooked at sea within hours of being caught, while "fresh" fish on the fishmonger's slab may be 2-3 weeks old.

Generally speaking it is vitamin C that suffers most in cooking and processing, and to a lesser extent vitamin B_1 in some foods; there is also a small loss in the quality of the protein. Garden-fresh foods are the best, frozen foods next best, then tinned foods; dried foods, on average, probably are least good. But the main loss is of vitamin C—there is no need to worry about the other nutrients.

Balancing losses against advantages

The main advantage of processing foods is that they are preserved (by canning, freezing, salting or drying) and will then keep for months or years. It means we can get foods all year around and from all countries. So even if processing does cause some loss of nutrients, at least we do get the food. In fact, it would be quite impossible without food-processing to feed the large numbers of people living in cities; so in some cases it is not a question of processed food versus fresh food, but processed food versus no food whatever.

There are also health advantages, such as in the pasteurization of milk. Although pasteurization destroys about a quarter of the vitamin C in milk and a tenth of the vitamins B_1, B_6, B_{12} and folic acid, this is a price worth paying for the safety from disease that can occur from drinking raw, untreated milk. More modern methods, such as selling sterilized milk in cardboard containers, suffer about the same loss but make milk available to many people, especially children, who would not otherwise get any.

Certainly not all food manufacturers pay attention to the nutritional value of their products, and many processed foods could be of higher nutritional quality if they were more carefully made or better methods of processing were used. At the same time, not all cooks are angels in the kitchen: some of them damage both the nutritional quality and the taste of foods far more than any manufacturer would ever dare do, for he would not be able to sell the products that are inflicted on some families.

SOME MYTHS

The recent interest in food and health has given rise to numerous articles in the press, and to radio and television programmes, not all of which present the facts correctly. This publicity has given rise to several modern myths.

Convenience foods These are blamed for many, if not all, of our modern ills, from dental decay and obesity to constipation and cancer. In fact, convenience foods, as such, are not to blame for anything, because the term simply means foods that have been partly or largely prepared for us by the manufacturer.

Bread was one of the earliest convenience foods. The manufacturer saves us the trouble of making it ourselves, it can be used for many purposes, it is easily carried about and keeps fairly well. In fact, wholemeal bread is generally regarded as being a very "healthy" food. When wheat is milled to white flour to make the white bread that many people prefer, part of the nutrients are lost—but that is a different matter.

In the same way, anything canned or bottled is ready to eat without further preparation apart perhaps from warming. Such convenience foods can be, although they are not always, as good as the same foods cooked at home; depending on the cook, they can taste better or worse, and can be nutritionally better or worse, than those made at home. Each food and each process would have to be considered individually.

Fast foods Technically-speaking these are foods that can be prepared quickly on a large scale, and retail outlets therefore specialize in only a few foods instead of offering the larger menu that one expects in a restaurant. An early version of these fast-food outlets was the old fish-and-chip shop, followed later by shops specially selling chicken, pizzas or hamburgers.

As regards nutrients, they are similar to the same thing produced at home; after all, a hamburger is only chopped-up meat. The criticism often made of hamburgers and some other fast-food products is that they are relatively rich in fat and salt. What we do not know is whether they contain more fat and salt than would the same dish prepared at home; presumably, if customers demanded, they could be "improved" in this respect.

In any manufactured product, of course, cheaper ingredients may be used. For example, it is most unlikely that any manufactured fish cake will contain as much fish as a housewife would use, simply because it would cost too much. In the same way, a meat product might contain more fat, or a fish finger more batter or breadcrumbs, than the equivalent food made at home. On the other hand, some people prefer their fish with batter....

Junk foods This is a term that has been applied to any food which is considered by the particular speaker or writer to be inferior. Scientifically the term means foods that supply energy and very little else; sugar and sweets supply energy without any nutrients, but any food in which the sugar content is high and the nutrients proportionately low would fall into this class.

The American *World Book Dictionary*, on the other hand, defines junk food as: "Ready-made or quickly prepared food, as that available in vending machines and fast-food establishments." The term "junk food", then, seems to have become a derogatory term—yet the nutritional value and taste of such foods can be, and often is, as good as that which "mother makes"; and if mother is a poor cook, they can be better.

Frozen foods These are subjected to much less treatment than any other process except for simple chilling or refrigeration. The freezing process itself and subsequent storage have no ultimate effect on nutritional value, but they have to be preceded by a blanching process—a few minutes' hot-water treatment—to destroy the enzymes naturally present, which would otherwise continue to function during frozen storage and thus spoil the food. This short cooking process washes out a small amount (depending on the size of the pieces of food) of the water-soluble nutrients, of which only vitamin C is of any importance.

However, since frozen foods are already partly cooked, they need less cooking at home than fresh foods do, and the combined effect of processing and shorter cooking time has been shown to be about the same as the longer cooking needed for fresh foods.

There is no nutritional change during frozen storage provided temperature is kept down to $0°F$ ($-18°C$), but there can be a further loss while the food is being thawed. But because the manufacturer almost always starts with fresher fruits and vegetables than the housewife can obtain from the shops, and because these therefore contain more vitamin C, frozen meals can actually have more vitamin C than a freshly cooked meal.

Microwave cooking Microwave cookers make use of electromagnetic radiation which quickly generates heat throughout the bulk of the food. This contrasts with conventional cooking where heat is applied to the surface of the food and has to be conducted into the inner parts.

The term "radiation"—although heat is itself infra-red radiation—sometimes causes concern about microwave cooking. There is absolutely no cause for worry unless the cooker itself is in such poor condition that the door fits badly so that radiation can leak out.

Irradiation The latest technique for treating food is by ionizing irradiation, of the same type as X-ray. Although the process sounds dangerous because the radiation usually comes from radioactive cobalt, it is in no way harmful. A food cooked in an electric oven is hardly likely to electrocute the consumer; it is equally wrong to suppose that ionizing radiation will make the food itself radioactive. The process has been thoroughly investigated for more than 20 years and internationally declared safe.

It has proved to be of value in eliminating the hazard of food-poisoning, by destroying the bacteria without affecting the food itself. It is particularly useful in preventing salmonella-poisoning from frozen poultry, which is an extremely common problem. Small doses kill off insects that infest stored grain, prevent fruits and vegetables from going mouldy, and prevent stored potatoes from sprouting.

It is therefore a most useful innovation. Yet surprisingly there is nothing new about this "latest" advance. X-rays were discovered in 1895, and as long ago as 1896 it was suggested that irradiation could be used to destroy bacteria in food. The process itself was patented half a century ago, but it is only now being permitted in a large number of countries.

Health foods and special diets

The term "health foods" is popularly applied to a large variety of foods and dietary practices, ranging from ones of excellent nutritional quality to ones which at best are of very doubtful value. Some practical preoccupations of "health food" adherents are discussed below.

"NATURAL" FOODS

In recent years many people, especially town dwellers, have found great pleasure—and fresh food—in growing their own crops. This has led to exaggerated claims for anything that is "natural", a fact that advertisers have not been slow to spot. We even have the ludicrous situation where margarine is advertised as being made from natural oils in opposition to claims that butter is natural. Natural vitamins—those extracted from foods—are more highly prized and consequently more highly priced than those made in a factory. In fact, the synthetic vitamin has to be identical in all respects with the natural one and possesses all its biological functions.

CHEMICAL ADDITIVES

As discussed earlier, the greater part of all our food is processed; almost the only foods that we eat fresh are some fruits and vegetables at certain seasons of the year. Processing includes the addition of a large number of chemicals as preservatives, for colouring, flavouring and many other purposes. Ready-peeled potatoes, for instance, are dipped into a solution of bisulphite to keep them from going brown, and this destroys some of their vitamin B_1—the price you pay for convenience. Sausages are preserved with sulphur dioxide as a safety measure in some countries, including the UK, and this destroys all the vitamin B_1, but this must be balanced against the possible health risk of untreated sausages.

Certainly colours are added to food for purely cosmetic reasons. This is what most people seem to want. Butter is coloured in the UK and elsewhere to standardize the colour all year, and so are fruit-juice drinks. The consumer has now been conditioned to believe that pale orange drinks must be low in fruit-juice content, that the grey colour of tinned garden peas makes them unpalatable, and that the brown colour of undyed strawberry jam is a mark of an inferior product.

There is currently no evidence that these additives do any harm, but neither is there evidence that they are perfectly safe. Some of the colourings used in foods are derived from plants and there is a tendency to assume that this makes them safer than the synthetic ones. In fact, this is quite incorrect. There are plenty of poisonous substances in nature and the natural additives are just as open to suspicion as any invented by man.

HOME-MADE FOODS

Health-food shops often stock home-made products in preference to factory-made ones. For example, many people like to buy home-made, hand-potted jam, which sometimes makes the additional claim of being cooked in copper pots. The appeal, of course, is a nostalgic one, for there is no reason at all for hand-potted jam to be superior to jam that enters the pot through a machine-controlled tap or valve—in fact, the factory jam may be potted more hygienically. Moreover, boiling the jam in copper pots destroys vitamin C very rapidly, while boiling in stainless steel does not.

On the other hand, if you make jam or marmalade yourself you may very well end up with a better product than a factory-made one. Most cooks can make jam, and certainly marmalade, that will set by using only fruit and sugar, whereas the commercial products are usually diluted with extra sugar because it is cheaper than fruit pulp and so need to have extra pectin added to make them set. So if the list of ingredients on the label includes pectin, it means that less fruit has been used and more sugar has been added. In fact many of the health-food, home-made, high-priced jams and marmalades also contain extra pectin, so there is no reason to assume that these are richer in fruit than the factory products.

Although extra fruit may make a great deal of difference to the taste it will make very little difference to nutritional value, providing only a little extra vitamin C.

A cake which you have made yourself might be nutritionally superior to a factory product, because the manufacturer would use, say, fewer eggs and less milk to keep prices down. But unless you know what has gone into a product, you cannot assume that the label "home-made" on produce in health-food shops guarantees that it has more value than factory produce.

"WHOLE FOODS"

Some health foods are described as "whole foods", meaning that they are unrefined or that no more has been removed from the plant than is necessary to make it edible. The foods in question are mainly cereal grains and brown sugar (although it should be noted that the outer part of oat bran, which has been used to polish metal, is not well tolerated by the human digestive tract). Whole grain and rice are certainly nutritionally preferable to white flour and polished rice, since they are richer in vitamins and iron, and very much richer in dietary fibre. Brown sugar, on the other hand, differs very little from white in its nutritional value. White sugar is 99.9-percent pure sucrose; brown 98-percent pure sucrose and 1-percent water; only the remaining 1 percent contains traces (but only traces) of vitamins and minerals. Treacle is a little less refined, but even so it contains only iron in any reasonable amount.

ORGANICALLY GROWN FOOD

While choosing to eat unprocessed or whole-grain foods creates no problems for other people, a widespread insistence on organically grown food would limit the amount of food that could be produced.

There is no evidence whatsoever that plants grown on soil organically manured by vegetable compost and animal droppings, and animals fed on such plants, are superior to those grown with or nourished on food grown with the aid of inorganic fertilizers such as sulphate of ammonia, phosphate and potash. In fact inorganic fertilizers are the *natural* food for plants, which take in their nutrients from the soil in the inorganic form supplied by nitrates, potassium salts and phosphates, and the trace elements. If, instead, they are supplied from an organic source such as rotted garden compost, animal manure, blood meal or hoof-and-horn meal (all of which are used by many gardeners) they must first be broken down in the soil to the relevant inorganic form before they can be absorbed by the plants.

It is true that organic material improves the texture and water-holding properties of the soil and that its nutrients are steadily released, but the latter can also be achieved by slow-release inorganic fertilizers. The best methods of cultivation would probably involve both organic and inorganic fertilizers, but this can be achieved only on a small scale. There is simply not enough organic material available to fertilize the vast areas of land needed to feed millions of people. If we did without inorganic fertilizers we would not produce enough food.

It is also argued that tractors compress the soil, that drips of tractor oil and fuel kill off earthworms, and that such ill-managed soil is less productive than organically manured soil untouched by the dead weight of a tractor. Even if this were true, it is difficult to visualize without these mechanical aids the vast Canadian wheatlands or the enormous areas in the USA where soya beans and corn are produced on such a gigantic scale that they feed populations around the world.

The same is true of the insecticides, herbicides and fungicides that are used on a vast scale in an attempt—not always successful—to protect crops from all their predators. Some have been pressed into use before being proved safe; but most countries now control the types of chemicals used and apply a limit to the amounts of such chemicals that may be left as residues in the food. Studies of our food have shown that the levels are very low, but obviously it would be preferable if they were non-existent. Unfortunately, this would once again severely curtail the amount of food produced.

VITAMIN SUPPLEMENTS

If you are getting enough vitamins in your diet, a supplement is not going to make you any healthier. There is no evidence to support the claims made for taking huge doses of vitamins ("megavitamin theory")—indeed, we know that vitamins A and D are toxic in large quantities. It may, however, be a good idea, and it will certainly do no harm, to take a small supplement (2 or 3 tablets of mixed vitamins a week) just in case your diet is deficient.

"MAGIC FOODS"

This category of health foods is a source of nonsense and profiteering. It sometimes seems that the principle is that a food must be very good for you if it is rarely eaten in your country. For example, buckwheat is almost unknown in the UK outside pet-food shops, but it is highly regarded by some health-food devotees. In Canada and the USA it is an ordinary vegetable, so commonly eaten that there is little point in making a speciality of it, and in central Europe it is the food of the peasants. That may make it very ordinary or very special, depending on your point of view.

Similarly, when yogurt was little known in the West it gained a special esteem. There were stories of Balkan peasants who lived to the magical age of 107 through eating it. Now that yogurt has become a very common food it has lost its "magical" properties—unless, of course, it is "live" yogurt instead of pasteurized "dead" material; then it regains its properties, we are told.

Honey occupies a special place in food mythology, possibly because of its unique source and because it has been known for so many thousands of years. It has been claimed to cure a multitude of disorders from tiredness to baldness, to secure sexual virility and to confer tallness. In fact it is simply a solution of sugars (glucose and fructose) together with a very small trace of some vitamins and minerals—not enough to make it into a reasonable food even if eaten in large quantities. It has an attractive taste, depending on the flowers that the bees browsed on, but it has no special properties that sugar—white sugar at that—does not have.

Seaweed, especially kelp, is sold in health-food shops as particularly beneficial, although there is not a trace of evidence that it has any value other than as a source of iodine. Sea salt, which contains iodine but also traces of all the impurities of seawater, is sold at a very much higher price than the pure salt obtained on land.

Another delightful oddity is bee's royal jelly, once well described as "this b... nonsense". It is claimed to have rejuvenating qualities, and so instantly appeals to all of us who cannot otherwise prevent ourselves growing older—so long as we can afford the extremely high price. Since this is the food that transforms a worker bee into a queen bee, it must clearly be very good for human beings. The only problem—glossed over in the claims—is that a bee is very small: if you multiply the bee's dose by the relative weight of an adult you would need to eat 20 tons a day—assuming that you wanted to be transformed into a queen bee.

PILLS AND POTIONS

Products for sale in health-food shops often include pills, potions, and sometimes even charms with far-reaching and untenable claims. These products are sometimes made from herbs and flowers that have been thought over the centuries to be beneficial for some disorders, but there is no evidence that they have any effect whatever—except, maybe, through faith in them. Such products are often bought in the same way that lucky charms or witches' blessings were bought centuries ago—and if people believe that something will do them good it may actually help them.

Among the "cures" are simple salts that, taken in the "right" combination, alleviate, if they do not cure, aches, pains, discharges of the ears, and a host of other disorders. You may wonder why people should pay for tablets made from simple salts, but the answer is that they are not described in simple terms. For example, everyone knows that table salt is cheap and available in every kitchen, and many people know that the chemical name is sodium chloride, but very few know that the old name is natrium muriate. So people pay good money for "natrium muriate" without knowing that they are already consuming more of this than is good for them. Similarly, no one would pay for sand (except to mix with cement), but call it "silicon dioxide" and it assumes a special function. So does plaster of Paris when called "calcium sulphate".

Such "cures" are not merely misleading but can also be dangerous, since their existence suggests that self-treatment is preferable to taking medical advice.

VEGETARIANISM

Meat-eaters tend to believe that meat is essential for "strength" and that one cannot live without it. This is not true; in fact, in some respects, a vegetarian is eating a better diet than a meat-eater. If, as discussed earlier, one of the errors of our Western diets is that we eat too much saturated fat, then the vegetarian is eating a better diet, since most of our saturated fat comes from meat. Again, dietary fibre is beneficial, and most vegetarians are eating whole-grain cereals, which contain a great deal of dietary fibre. Finally, as already pointed out, it is a good idea to eat a wide variety of foods in order to make sure of getting all the nutrients that we need; because vegetarians are more interested in diet than most people they do tend to eat a wider variety of foods, especially of fruits, vegetables, nuts and legumes, even if their diet is restricted by losing out on the nutrients present in meat, poultry and fish.

So far as we know, the health of vegetarians is as good as that of most other people. They would claim that it is better.

Meat is certainly an excellent source of protein, of iron that is well absorbed and of a range of vitamins of the B group, but there are plenty of people in the world living, by necessity if not from choice, on a vegetarian diet.

VEGANISM

A vegan diet excludes anything that comes from an animal, so milk, eggs, butter and cheese are not eaten, nor is meat, fish and poultry. Vegans appear to maintain good health on their diet, but it is much more difficult to follow than vegetarianism and its success depends on knowing a fair amount about nutrition.

MACROBIOTIC DIET

Among the more esoteric diets is the Zen macrobiotic diet, which originated in the United States and is concerned with spiritual awakening or rebirth. It has been publicly criticized by the American Medical Association, firstly because the diet is supposed to replace all medical treatment and, secondly, because as the stages of the diet progress it becomes increasingly restricted and there is therefore the danger of incurring serious nutritional deficiencies. There have been many victims of such deficiencies and even some deaths caused by this diet in the USA.

Obesity and slimming

One of the most common, most talked about and most ignored problems of nutrition is obesity—most common because a quarter to a third (some reports say half) of the population of all industrialized countries is overweight; most talked about and most ignored because obese people tend to talk about their problem but do little else.

CAUSES OF OBESITY

We don't really know the true cause of obesity, but we do know that anyone gaining weight is eating more food energy than he or she is using up in activity. That is a simple statement of fact. What we do not know is why some people eat more food than they use up and why some people can eat large quantities without getting fat.

Earlier, Table 3 (page 18) showed a balance sheet for an office worker who consumed 2,620 Calories (11 megajoules) per day as food and spent about the same amount of energy in activity, so maintaining constant weight. If his body functioned mechanically (and in this sense some people's bodies do) and he ate one more slice of bread and butter a day, he would gain weight. A slice of bread and butter provides about 100 Calories (420 kilojoules) per day, which would amount to 10lb (4.5kg) of fat in a year. If this happened between the ages of 20 and 40 the extra daily slice of bread and butter could make him gain 200lb (90kg): he would at the age of 40 weigh $2\frac{1}{2}$ times what he weighed at twenty.

How then is it that at least half the population do not gain or lose weight? Can they really eat exactly the amount of energy they use? The fat office-worker ate only 100 Calories (420 kilojoules) extra per day, and gained 200lb (90kg); if he ate 10 Calories (42 kilojoules) extra he would, at the same rate, gain 20lb (9kg). Ten Calories (42 kilojoules) is one-tenth of a slice of bread and butter, or a few crumbs at each meal. Do people who maintain constant body weight really control their appetites to within a few crumbs a day?

The answer seems to be that some people, the ones whose weight stays the same for years on end, adjust their energy output to match their food intake, not the other way around. In other words, they burn off any surplus they have eaten, while their less fortunate friends are much more efficient and keep, as fat, all the extra food they eat. Some people appear to function like a savings bank—energy in minus energy out equals gain (or loss) of weight. Others are apparently born with a different mechanism, and whatever they eat they somehow keep their weight constant.

Then there are people who really do eat greedily, never leaving the table while there is food still on it. Most of these people will get fat, but why do they behave in this way? The behavioural scientists have been looking closely at such people during the last few years and conclude that they "eat with their eyes". The sight of food appears to act as a trigger to make them feel hungry; when they don't see it they don't feel hungry. The appetite of more "normal" people does not depend on seeing food.

People who say, "Why can she eat [it is usually she] twice as much as me and stay as skinny as a rail while I eat very little and every ounce stays on?" are sometimes not being quite truthful about their own eating habits. However, it is true that some people are born with small requirements; that is, a low metabolic rate. The average adult man, for example, who is moderately active eats about 2,500-3,000 Calories (10-12 megajoules) a day. If his weight does not change he must be using this amount. But some men of the same size and age, and doing the same work, may need only 2,000 Calories (8 megajoules), and so would get fat on a diet of 3,000 Calories (12 megajoules). Yet others need 4,000 Calories (16 megajoules): people really do differ as much as this, and even more. So a person with a lower metabolic rate (meaning simply that he or she burns off energy at a lower rate) will get fat even by eating only normal portions of food.

HOW FAT IS TOO FAT?

Despite all these different factors it is still true that anyone gaining weight is taking in more than they are using, and anyone who is currently fat must have done that at some time. But how fat is "fat"—and what is "excess weight"?

Firstly, it is fat, or adipose tissue, that we are really talking about, not weight. People can be heavier than average, but not fat, if they develop large muscles. Weight, however, is almost always a useful guide to body fat.

Secondly, people differ a great deal from one another in every respect, including their "ideal" body-weight, but the best we can do is to compare them with the *average* weight. It has been shown by insurance company statistics that people of average body-weight, or slightly less, live longer than those who are 12lb (6kg) or more above average weight. The heavier you are the shorter life you can expect. Men who are 10-percent overweight have a 13-percent increased death risk. This rises to 25 percent if they are 20-percent overweight and to 42 percent if they are 30-percent overweight. For women the increased death risk is 9 percent, 21 percent and 30 percent for each of the stages of fatness.

Put another way, a man over 45 who is 25lb (12kg) overweight reduces his life expectancy by 25 percent: he is likely to die at 60 instead of 80. Studies have shown that if he loses his surplus fat he greatly reduces the risk. These, of course, are averages; some fat people live a long time (and some thin people die young).

Fat people have increased risk of diabetes, and high blood pressure with the many disorders that this gives rise to: heart disease, bronchitis, gallstones, varicose veins and diseased joints. They are at greater risk in surgery and in childbirth and have a higher accident rate.

How do you know if you are too fat? Tables 19-21 show the acceptable range of weights for a given height, the middle weight in each range being the one recommended for good health. Anyone exceeding the upper limit is considered overweight, and obesity is defined as 20 percent more than the upper limit.

Some weight tables and weighing machines carry "desirable" weights for people of different frame sizes. As it is difficult to assess frame size, the various authorities have dropped any mention of them from their tables and give instead an "acceptable weight range"—as here.

LOSING WEIGHT

So what can be done? Everyone knows the answer to that. If gaining weight is caused by taking in more energy than you use, then taking in less energy than you use (which is not necessarily the same as taking in less food) will cause you to lose weight.

Crash or fad diets—banana diets, grapefruit diets and so on—are not much use because as soon as you stop them you will put on weight again. The same is true of drugs, which may also have undesirable side-effects.

Fasting is certainly not to be recommended unless it is done under medical supervision. Firstly, it is dangerous because in addition to fat some of the more essential parts of the body such as the tissues themselves may be used up, causing serious damage. Secondly, the body needs nutrients all the time and by fasting you would be depriving yourself of essential proteins, vitamins and minerals. And lastly, while a short fast of a few days would certainly use up some fat, this shares the disadvantage of crash diets in that you would probably resume the eating habits that made you fat in the first place.

What about exercise? If energy in minus energy out equals energy left in the body, then you should be able to lose weight by increasing energy expenditure. In practice, though, you have to exercise an awful lot to lose 2 lb (1 kg) of fat. It would take a 100-mile walk.

Suppose you decide to walk a fast mile or so every night after dinner instead of slumping in front of the television set. You would lose only about one-fifteenth of an ounce (2 g) of weight. And if you stop at the bar on the way back don't have more than half a pint of beer, otherwise you will gain weight. It should also be remembered that exercise might give you a greater appetite.

(cont'd on page 60)   55

19 Desirable weights for adults*

MEN

Height		Weights in lb		
ft in	lower	average	upper	obese
5 2	112	123	141	169
5 3	115	127	144	173
5 4	118	130	148	178
5 5	121	133	152	182
5 6	124	136	156	187
5 7	128	140	161	193
5 8	132	145	166	199
5 9	136	149	170	204
5 10	140	153	174	209
5 11	144	158	179	215
6 0	148	162	184	221
6 1	152	166	189	227
6 2	156	171	194	233
6 3	160	176	199	239
6 4	164	181	204	245

Height m		Weights in kg		
1.58	51	55.8	64	77
1.60	52	57.6	65	78
1.62	53	58.6	66	79
1.64	54	59.6	67	80
1.66	55	60.6	69	83
1.68	56	61.7	71	85
1.70	58	63.5	73	88
1.72	59	65.0	74	89
1.74	60	66.5	75	90
1.76	62	68.0	77	92
1.78	64	69.4	79	95
1.80	65	71.0	80	96
1.82	66	72.6	82	98
1.84	67	74.2	84	101
1.86	69	75.8	86	103
1.88	71	77.6	88	106
1.90	73	79.3	90	108
1.92	75	81.0	93	112

*Weights given without clothes. For indoor clothing, add: men 7-9lb (3-4kg), women 4-6lb (2.25kg). Lower and upper weights are acceptable limits for each height.

WOMEN

| Height | | Weights in lb | | |
ft in	lower	average	upper	obese
4 10	92	102	119	143
4 11	94	104	122	146
5 0	96	107	125	150
5 1	99	110	128	154
5 2	102	113	131	157
5 3	105	116	134	161
5 4	108	120	138	166
5 5	111	123	142	170
5 6	114	128	146	175
5 7	118	132	150	180
5 8	122	136	154	185
5 9	126	140	158	190
5 10	130	144	163	196
5 11	134	148	168	202
6 0	138	152	173	208

Height m		Weights in kg		
	lower	average	upper	obese
1.45	42	46.0	53	64
1.48	42	46.5	54	65
1.50	43	47.0	55	66
1.52	44	48.5	57	68
1.54	44	49.5	58	70
1.56	45	50.4	58	70
1.58	46	51.3	59	71
1.60	48	52.6	61	73
1.62	49	54.0	62	74
1.64	50	55.4	64	77
1.66	51	56.8	65	78
1.68	52	58.1	66	79
1.70	53	60.0	67	80
1.72	55	61.3	69	83
1.74	56	62.6	70	84
1.76	58	64.0	72	86
1.78	59	65.3	74	89

20 Height/weight/age table for boys of school age

Age	Heights in inches			Weights in lb		
	lower	average	upper	lower	average	upper
6	42	45	48	37	45	53
7	45	47	50	42	50	60
8	47	50	53	47	55	67
9	49	52	55	51	60	73
10	51	54	57	55	65	82
11	53	56	59	62	73	90
12	55	58	61	68	82	102
13	57	60	63	71	90	112
14	60	63	67	88	108	133
15	63	66	70	105	126	152
16	65	68	71	112	133	160
17	65	69	72	118	137	165

21 Height/weight/age table for girls of school age

Age	Heights in inches			Weights in lb		
	lower	average	upper	lower	average	upper
6	42	44	47	37	44	53
7	44	47	50	42	50	60
8	46	49	52	44	53	64
9	48	51	54	46	56	68
10	50	53	56	53	64	79
11	52	55	58	62	73	90
12	55	58	61	68	84	105
13	57	60	64	75	93	117
14	60	62	66	88	108	132
15	61	65	68	100	123	148
16	61	65	68	108	128	154
17	61	65	68	110	130	157

Age	Heights in cm			Weights in kg		
	lower	average	upper	lower	average	upper
6	108	115	122	17	20	24
7	113	120	128	19	22	27
8	119	127	134	21	25	30
9	124	132	139	23	27	33
10	129	137	145	25	30	37
11	134	142	150	28	33	41
12	139	147	155	30	37	46
13	144	152	160	32	40	51
14	152	161	170	40	49	60
15	160	169	178	47	57	68
16	164	173	181	51	60	72
17	166	175	183	53	62	74

Age	Heights in cm			Weights in kg		
	lower	average	upper	lower	average	upper
6	106	113	120	17	20	24
7	112	119	127	19	22	27
8	117	125	132	20	24	29
9	122	130	137	21	26	31
10	127	135	143	24	29	36
11	132	140	148	28	33	41
12	140	148	156	31	38	47
13	146	154	162	34	42	53
14	150	158	167	40	49	60
15	155	164	173	46	56	67
16	155	164	173	49	58	70
17	155	164	173	50	59	71

Although it is not an efficient way of losing weight, however, exercise is a useful way of preventing a weight gain. A slice of bread and butter supplies enough energy for a brisk 10-minute walk. So if our fat office worker who gained 200 lb (90 kg) by eating one extra slice of bread and butter a day for 20 years had also walked an extra ten minutes a day he would not have gained weight at all. (This, of course, assumes that the body behaves like an accurate weighing machine, which it doesn't, but it is a rather good illustration of the value of exercise with regard to body fat.) Of course, exercise is essential for good health, and jogging seems to be beneficial in warding off heart problems even though it does not get rid of much fat.

But if you want to lose weight, and keep it off, the only real answer is to learn to eat sensibly, and to keep these new eating habits for life.

HOW MUCH FOOD?

How much should you eat on a reducing diet? The important thing is to ensure that you are getting all the proteins, vitamins and minerals that you need without getting also too much energy. If, for instance, you normally ate about 2,500 Calories (10 megajoules) per day and reduced this to 1,250 Calories (5 megajoules), you would also be halving your usual supply of proteins, vitamins and minerals; you would have to be very careful therefore in your choice of food to ensure you were getting an adequate supply of these nutrients.

Reducing diets are usually based on about 1,200-1,500 Calories (6 megajoules) per day. With this amount it is not difficult to select foods that are rich in nutrients and low in energy value: meat, poultry, fish, cottage cheese, plenty of fruit and vegetables.

Remember that it took a long time to gain weight, so don't expect to lose it all in a few weeks. The fat office worker took 20 years to gain 200 lb (90 kg); a less extreme case might take a year to gain about 22 lb (10 kg). Even if you ate nothing at all you would lose only 12 oz (0.34 kg) of weight a day.

If you were about 1,000 Calories (4 megajoules) short every day you could expect to lose about 1-2 lb (0.5-1 kg) every week (plus some water in the first week which would make the bathroom scales seem rather encouraging). Weight does not always fall steadily, but don't be discouraged—stick to it.

The main requirement for slimming is incentive and willpower. Do you really want to lose weight? No one can do it for you. If you find it difficult to reduce on your own you could join a slimming club, such as Weight Watchers, where you learn to eat sensibly. If you really must nibble between meals, try a nibble bowl of celery, cucumber, and radishes or green peppers.

WHAT IS BROWN FAT?

Some people can eat as much as they like and never gain weight. They seem to burn off any excess food as waste heat, but we are not certain how they do it.

There is a certain amount of "brown fat" in the body—ordinary fat is nearly white—which metabolizes faster than ordinary fat and produces more heat. It seems possible, although it remains to be proved, that people who do not gain weight have more brown fat than others. In any case, whatever the reason, there is nothing one can do about it, for anyone who is overweight has no alternative but to reduce their intake of calories.

DOES DIETARY FIBRE HELP?

It has been suggested that fibre-rich foods are a help in slimming, but this has never been tested. People have lost weight on a low-calorie diet rich in fibre but have not been tested on a low-calorie diet without any extra fibre.

Such a diet is worth trying, however, because fibre, in theory at least, might be helpful. It is possible that you might eat less because fibre-rich foods (such as wholemeal bread, as against white bread) take longer to chew, causing more saliva to be produced; the volume reaching the stomach is greater and you might therefore feel full on less food. Finally, fibre slows down the emptying of the stomach, and as a result you might not feel hungry so soon.

Theory aside, a useful way of eating the usual amount of food while reducing your calorie intake is to eat several helpings of fruits and vegetables every day. These are bulky, low-calorie foods which will supply minerals and vitamins while helping you to feel full.

CHILDREN AND WEIGHT

Because children are growing it is necessary to take both age and height into consideration when assessing their weight. Tables 20 and 21 (pages 58–59) are collected from a number of different sources which provide the range of heights and weights considered to be acceptable for each age. They can be used only as an approximate guide. As with the table for adults (Table 19), weights in excess of 10 percent and 20 percent above the upper limit are considered to be overweight and obese respectively.

Questions and answers

Q My child won't drink milk. Will he get enough calcium from other foods?

A You get the same amount of calcium, about 250mg, which is nearly one third a child's RDA, from a glass of milk, 1oz (30g) of cheddar cheese (cream cheese and curd cheese do not contain much calcium), a 5oz (140g) carton of yogurt, or 7 slices of enriched white bread. So if these are the "other foods", yes, he can get enough.

Q My nails are soft and split easily. Will eating gelatin help strengthen them?

A There is one report of what on paper seems to have been a well-conducted trial which shows that $\frac{1}{2}$oz (15g) of gelatin a day did help to strengthen fingernails. This has neither been confirmed nor disproved, so it is worth trying.

Q I have bad acne. Are there foods I should avoid?

A We don't really know—sugary foods may be a contributory cause and so should be avoided.

Q Is it true that sufferers from migraine should not eat cheese and chocolate?

A Many foods have been shown to be a cause of migraine in different people. While chocolate, cheese and red wine have often been blamed in the past, recent trials show that almost any food can cause the problem. Sufferers should note what they have been eating just before the pain comes on, and try to work out for themselves what foods to avoid.

Q Is it true that you should "starve a fever, feed a cold?"

A No. In fact, when you are running a fever you are burning off energy at double the normal rate, so you should actually feed a fever—even though you probably don't feel much like eating.

Q Should I take extra salt or salt tablets in a hot climate?

A If you are sweating profusely, yes. Water intake is also a major problem, although your own thirst usually makes you drink. But during the first few days in such a climate your thirst may be a bit late in telling you when to drink and the sweat loss may make you feel slightly sick and unable to eat. You should therefore drink a lot of fluid, any kind, whenever sweat losses are unusually large.

Q Do you need a special diet after certain illnesses—for example, after a heart attack?

A After any illness it is essential to restore the body's reserve of nutrients, so a nutrient-rich diet is necessary for several weeks. This can be achieved by cutting down our sugar and fats and replacing them with more complete, nourishing foods.

After a heart attack it is necessary to ensure that you are not at all overweight and to restrict fatty foods severely. To be on the safe side, cholesterol intake should be limited by keeping the number of eggs per week down to four or less. Cut down also on red meat; poultry has less cholesterol.

Q Can depression be helped by a change in diet?

A This is still the subject of research and no answer is available.

Q Can a mother pass on her eating habits to her baby during pregnancy?

A No, not so far as we know.

Q Should I change my eating habits during pregnancy?

A Depends on how bad they were before. You need a "balanced diet"—see below.

Q Is it true that nothing in itself is bad for you, but that some things are better for you than others?

A In small amounts nothing is bad for you, even alcohol. It is when you take abnormally large amounts of particular foods that they may themselves cause harm. They push the better foods out of the diet.

Q Does a large dose of vitamin C prevent a cold?

A Unfortunately, no. A few experiments suggest that doses of 1g or so of vitamin C might shorten a cold or lessen the symptoms, but there is no clear evidence.

NUTRITION

Q What is meant by a balanced diet?

A Simply a good diet, with enough of all the nutrients—protein, vitamins and mineral salts—rather than one overloaded with fat or carbohydrate and relatively short of many of these nutrients.

Q Is an irregular diet necessarily a bad thing?

A In theory the body should receive a regular supply of nutrients—three meals a day—but many people manage very well indeed on one meal a day or even when eating irregularly. Probably it would be better if they did eat regularly.

Q Is it true that if you are going to eat one big meal a day it ought to be breakfast so that you have time to burn it up during the day?

A It does not matter and is largely a matter of habit.

Q Is it true that you should not eat and drink together, that is, is it better to drink before (or after) a meal?

A It does not matter.

Q How much protein is good for you? Is it possible to eat too much protein?

A The amount of protein that we need is only about 6-7 percent of the diet, but that would not be very palatable. On average we consume about 12-15 percent of our food in the form of protein. Taking more, however, is neither good nor bad.

Q Why do some foods upset certain people?

A Some people are allergic to certain foods, either natural or processed, or to some food additives (such as the yellow colour, tartrazine, which can affect perhaps one person in every few thousand). Most other people are quite un-affected by these, so for the vast majority of people the additives are quite safe—and one could hardly ban meat, milk or tea, or whatever foods affect some people. They should find out which foods or which additives affect them and refrain from consuming them.

Q Is a varied diet better than a stable one? Wild animals, after all, live well on the same food all the time.

A In order to get all the nutrients we need we have to consume a large number of different foods, for no single food supplies all the necessary nutrients. People on mono-tonous diets sometimes suffer from nutritional defici-encies. Farm animals and our pets are usually fed a complete mixture containing all the required nutrients, especially nowadays when we know fairly exactly what nutrients they need. But even if we knew exactly what is required for our own good health we would hardly enjoy eating a packet of complete nutrients at every meal.

Q Is butter better than margarine?

A On the contrary, margarine is richer in vitamin D than butter because it is added by law; it is as rich as summer butter in vitamin A, and thus richer than winter butter; and special margarines are rich in polyunsaturated fatty acids, while butter is far more saturated.

Q Why is brown bread considered healthier than white?

A Because it contains more of the B vitamins, iron and dietary fibre. Enriched white bread is not as rich in these as wholemeal bread. Some brown breads are not much better than white, and others are close to wholemeal; the word "brown" covers a range of breads.

Q Why is brown rice better than white rice?
A White rice is made by milling the bran from brown rice, the rice germ being lost at the same time. This reduces the amount of B vitamins and fibre. Some specially prepared products fall in between, and in some countries (not the UK) white rice is enriched with B vitamins.

Q Is brown sugar better for you than white sugar?
A There is no measurable difference. Both are nearly 100-percent sucrose.

SLIMMING

Q How fat can you get?
A One of the fattest men ever was Britain's William Campbell who reached $53\frac{1}{2}$ stone—750lb or 340kg—in 1878.

This enormous weight gave him about 2 million Calories of surplus fat, but because he died at the age of 22 he could have built up this store by eating only 250 surplus Calories each day of his life.

Q Is it helpful to take weight-reducing drugs?
A For most people, no. There is a strong risk of side effects, and when they stop taking the drug they tend to return to the wrong eating habits that made them fat in the first place.

Q Will I lose weight if I exercise regularly?
A Usually, yes, but not much. See the section on losing weight in OBESITY AND SLIMMING.

Q Would skipping a meal help me to lose weight?
A No. Skipping meals usually results in eating more at the next meal—or between meals. Better to learn improved eating habits at all meals.

Q Will it help me to lose weight if I eat more slowly?
A No, but what it might do is make you eat less. If you overeat because you love food, slowly savouring each mouthful might lead to a smaller intake. But if you are fat because your needs are small then it will probably have no effect at all.

Q When slimming, should you avoid salt because it leads to water retention?
A In a healthy person, even if obese, water and salt balance themselves automatically, and the body contains a fairly constant amount of water. Extra salt simply causes more thirst and both are excreted. But generally we all eat too much salt.

Q Does constipation make you fat?
A No: it might cause a bulge but it does not make any fatty tissue.

Q Will I put on weight if I give up smoking?
A Many people put on weight when they stop smoking. For some people this is because they eat more, because smoking depresses the appetite and tends to spoil the taste of food. But even if you do not eat any more you may still gain weight because smoking has some effect in speeding up the metabolism and burning up food a little faster.

Q How can you measure your metabolism, and can it be altered?
A Metabolism can easily be measured in the laboratory or hospital, but unfortunately it cannot be altered. Some people are unluckily born with a slow metabolic rate, so they need only, say, 1,500 Calories a day compared to the average of about 2,300. They would actually gain weight on the average diet, and even on an ordinary reducing diet. Others are born with the ability to burn off any extra food they eat.

Q Are there any special slimming foods? Is it true that a grapefruit before a meal will burn up the carbohydrate?
A No food is reducing. Some foods supply less energy than others, so it does help to replace energy-dense foods that contain sugar or fats with low-energy foods, such as vegetables and many fruits.

There is nothing in the idea of the grapefruit diet—or the potato diet, pineapple diet or any other similar fad.

Recipes for better health

Recipe books are usually intended to improve cooking skills and add to the variety of the diet. Here we provide a selection of recipes that should achieve both these objectives while at the same time improving the diet nutritionally.

Some of the recipes are:
low in fat—marked ●
low in salt—marked ▲
low in sugar—marked ■

Very often a reduction in fat and sugar will automatically reduce calorie-intake, because these two ingredients are concentrated energy.

It is easy to plan an attractive, palatable diet that fulfils the desired nutritional goals (see pages 22-23). It is a matter of selecting the right foods while reducing the amount of wrong foods, and using recipes that point in this direction. Weight reduction and "healthy eating" need be neither painful nor unappetizing.

Low-fat spreads, low-fat cheese and low-fat milk (which is 2-percent fat, instead of 4-percent as in full-cream milk) as well as skimmed milk are widely available, and can help to reduce energy and fat intake. While it is true that low-fat spreads are simply ordinary margarine-type fats with added water and air so that they collapse when heated, they are useful for sautéing because the water in the spread helps to cover the food.

Many standard recipes can be improved nutritionally by simply reducing the amounts of sugar and fat, and proportionately increasing the other ingredients. Similarly the salt can often be reduced: salting food is largely a matter of habit.

Hors d'oeuvre

CHICKEN-LIVER PÂTÉ

4oz (110g) chicken livers
2oz (60g) onion, chopped
1 egg, hard-boiled
Pinch of salt; pepper to taste
1 teaspoon low-fat spread

Place the livers and onion in a saucepan with one tablespoon of water. Cook gently until tender. Drain well, add salt and pepper, and mince together with the egg. Add the

67

low-fat spread, mash well with a fork and serve cold on a bed of lettuce.

Calories per serving: 130   **Serves 2**

MACKEREL PÂTÉ

4oz (110g) smoked mackerel fillets
½ garlic clove, crushed
Black pepper to taste
2 teaspoons lemon juice
1oz (30g) low-fat yogurt

Skin fillets, chop roughly, add other ingredients and pound well until soft.

Calories per serving: 120   **Serves 2**

"FRENCH" MUSHROOMS ● ▲

4oz (110g) button mushrooms
1oz (30g) low-fat spread
1 garlic clove, crushed
Dash of black pepper

Place all the ingredients in a small pan, bring to the boil, stirring well, cover and cook gently until tender (about 6 minutes). Serve at once.

Calories per serving: 55   **Serves 2**

PRAWNS IN TOMATOES

4 large tomatoes
4oz (110g) peeled cooked prawns
2 tablespoons low-calorie salad cream
4 tablespoons tinned sweetcorn
Salt and pepper
Lettuce leaves, finely shredded

Cut the tops off the tomatoes and set them aside. Using a metal teaspoon, scoop the insides out of the tomatoes, being careful to keep the shells intact. Discard the insides. Mix the prawns, salad cream, corn, salt and pepper together and pile the mixture into the tomato shells. Replace the tomato tops. Arrange on shredded lettuce. Serve chilled.

Calories per serving: 130   **Serves 2**

PRAWN SURPRISE ●

8 large Pacific prawns, cooked and peeled
8 lettuce leaves
¼ garlic clove, crushed
2 tablespoons white wine vinegar

Red and yellow peppers (capsicum), thinly sliced

Mix the vinegar and garlic together. Roll each prawn in a lettuce leaf, place 4 on each plate, garnish with the sliced peppers and pour the garlic vinegar over them.

Calories per serving: 30　　　　　　　　　　　**Serves 2**

MOULES MARINIÈRES ●

12fl.oz (340ml) dry white wine
4fl.oz (110ml) water
2 garlic cloves, crushed
2 tablespoons chopped fresh parsley
2 bay leaves
4 tomatoes, chopped
Pepper
24 large mussels

Put all the ingredients except the mussels in a shallow pan. Cover the pan and bring the liquid to the boil. Reduce the heat and simmer for 5 minutes. Meanwhile, scrub the mussels clean and tug out the "beards". Give them a final rinse in a large bowl of cold water and drain well. Remove the pan from the heat and pour the liquid through a strainer. Discard the contents of the strainer and return the liquid to the shallow pan. Arrange the mussels in the pan and cover. Steam over moderate heat for about 6 minutes until they open. Discard any mussels which have not opened. Serve immediately.

Calories per serving: 260　　　　　　　　　　**Serves 2**

For more hors d'oeuvre ideas, see the section on Salads.

Soups

WATERCRESS AND YOGURT SOUP ● ▲

2 large bunches watercress, chopped
½ pint (3dl) water
½ pint (3dl) low-fat natural yogurt
Pepper

Put the watercress and water into a saucepan and simmer for 15 minutes. Blend the contents in a blender, or rub them through a strainer, and return to the pan. Stir in the yogurt, add pepper to taste, reheat over low heat and serve.

Calories per serving: 75　　　　　　　　　　　**Serves 2**

CONSOMMÉ WITH VEGETABLES ●

1 tin consommé (beef or chicken)

2 medium carrots, diced
1 medium leek, finely chopped
2 tomatoes, chopped
Salt and pepper

Put all the ingredients except the salt and pepper into a saucepan and simmer, covered, over low heat until the vegetables are tender but not mushy. Taste the soup and if necessary add salt and pepper. Serve hot.

Calories per serving: 20   **Serves 2**

LEEK AND TOMATO SOUP ●▲

2 large leeks, finely chopped
2 large tomatoes, chopped
1 bay leaf
Pinch of dried mixed herbs
5fl.oz (140ml) water
5fl.oz (140ml) low-fat natural yogurt
Pepper

Put the vegetables, herbs and water into a saucepan and simmer, covered, until the vegetables are tender. Discard the bay leaf and blend the mixture in a blender, or rub it through a strainer. Return the soup to the pan, and stir in the yogurt and pepper to taste. Reheat over low heat and serve.

Calories per serving: 50   **Serves 2**

CELERY SOUP ●

15oz (450g) tin of celery, well drained
1 pint (½ litre) low-fat milk
Salt and pepper to taste
Large sprig of parsley

Blend celery and milk, season to taste, heat gently to boiling point and serve sprinkled with parsley.

Calories per serving: 100   **Serves 2**

Egg and cheese dishes

BASIC OMELET

4 small eggs
Pepper
2 tablespoons water
½oz (15g) butter

Beat the eggs, pepper and water together. Heat the butter over moderate heat in an omelet pan, swirling it around so that it coats the bottom of the pan. Pour in the beaten eggs and stir lightly with a fork for the first few seconds. When the bottom of the omelet is beginning to set, lift up one edge with a spatula and tip the runny egg in that direction. Put the pan straight over the flame again and, if you like, sprinkle with a filling (see below). When the omelet is cooked, flip it over quickly with a spatula so that it is folded in half. Serve immediately on a hot plate.

Calories per serving: 200   Serves 2

OMELET FILLINGS

Even with the fillings the omelets are still low in calories.

Chicken
4oz (110g) diced cooked chicken
4 spring onions, finely shredded
Calories per serving: 290   Serves 2

Fines herbes
2 teaspoons each fresh chopped
parsley, thyme and tarragon
Calories per serving: 200   Serves 2

Cheese and tomato
2 large tomatoes, finely chopped
2oz (60g) low-fat cheese, grated
Calories per serving: 290   Serves 2

Mushroom
4oz (110g) button mushrooms, halved,
poached and drained
1 shallot, very finely sliced
Calories per serving: 210   Serves 2

Beef and asparagus
4oz (110g) lean beef, diced
4 sticks asparagus, fresh and chopped,
or tinned without added salt
Calories per serving: 250   Serves 2

Prawn
4oz (110g) peeled cooked prawns
4 teaspoons chopped fresh chives
Calories per serving: 260   Serves 2

SPANISH OMELET

3 tablespoons butter
2 shallots (or 1 small onion), finely chopped
1 tinned pimiento, chopped
4oz (110g) cooked green beans, chopped
4oz (110g) button mushrooms, halved
Pepper
4 eggs

Melt 2 tablespoons of the butter in a saucepan, and add the vegetables and pepper. Fry gently until the vegetables are cooked. Remove the pan from the heat. Melt the remaining butter in an omelet pan. Beat the eggs and a little pepper together with a fork and pour them into the omelet pan. Stir the eggs lightly with a fork until the bottom of the omelet is just beginning to set. Sprinkle the vegetables over the top of the omelet and serve when the egg has set.

Calories per serving: 360   **Serves 2**

LEMON SOUFFLÉ OMELET

4 eggs, separated
Juice and finely grated rind of 2 large lemons
Liquid sweetener to taste
1 tablespoon butter

Put the egg yolks, lemon juice and rind, and sweetener in a bowl. Beat well with a fork, then beat the egg whites until stiff, and using a metal spoon, fold in. Melt the butter in an omelet pan and pour in the mixture. Cook over low heat until the bottom has set and looks lightly browned. Remove the pan from the heat and hold it under a moderately hot grill until the top is browned and set. The middle should be slightly runny. Serve immediately.

Calories per serving: 210   **Serves 2**

SCRAMBLED EGGS WITH ASPARAGUS

4 eggs
Pepper
$\frac{1}{2}$ teaspoon paprika
2 tablespoons water
12 large asparagus spears, steamed
$\frac{1}{2}$oz (15g) butter, melted

Beat the eggs, salt, pepper, paprika and water together with a fork. Scramble over moderate heat in a saucepan. Put the scrambled egg on a warmed plate. Lay the asparagus spears down beside the egg, pour the melted butter over and serve.

Calories per serving: 230   **Serves 2**

HUEVOS FLAMENCOS ▲

4 eggs
1oz (30g) fresh or frozen peas
1oz (30g) frozen or tinned (unsweetened) sweetcorn
1oz (30g) precooked or frozen carrots, diced
Black pepper to taste
Small quantity of low-fat spread

Take 2 fairly shallow ovenproof dishes, large enough to

allow the eggs to spread out, and grease the dishes sparsely with the low-fat spread. Break 2 eggs into each dish, keeping the yolks whole. Sprinkle half the vegetables onto each dish and shake on a little pepper. Bake in a moderate oven (350°F/180°C) until the whites are hard and the yolks just set. Serve hot.

Calories per serving: 170   **Serves 2**

SCRAMBLED EGGS WITH SMOKED SALMON

4 eggs
1 tablespoon chopped fresh chives
2 tablespoons milk
4oz (110g) smoked salmon, cut into thin strips

Beat the eggs, chives and milk together and put them in a saucepan. Scramble over low heat. When the eggs are nearly scrambled, stir in the smoked salmon. Serve hot.

Calories per serving: 260   **Serves 2**

MACARONI CHEESE ●▲

4oz (110g) macaroni
¾ pint (4dl) skimmed milk
¾oz (20g) margarine
1oz (30g) plain flour
4oz (110g) low-fat cheese

Boil the macaroni and drain off the water. Make white sauce from the milk, flour and margarine (see Basic sauces, page 80). Add ¾ of the cheese, then the macaroni, sprinkle the rest of the cheese on top and brown under the grill.

Calories per serving: 370   **Serves 3**

CAULIFLOWER CHEESE ●▲

½ small cauliflower (about 12oz/340g)
¼ pint (140ml) skimmed milk
⅓oz (10g) margarine
½oz (15g) plain flour
2oz (60g) low-fat cheese, grated
Pinch of pepper

Boil the cauliflower until tender, drain, retaining about 1½ fl.oz (50ml) of the water, and keep the cauliflower hot. Make a white sauce from the flour, margarine, and cauliflower water topped up with the milk (see Basic sauces, page 80). Add ¾ of the cheese, with pepper to season, and pour over the cauliflower. Sprinkle the remaining grated cheese over the top, and brown under the grill.

Calories per serving: 160   **Serves 2**

Meat, poultry and fish dishes

SLIMMER'S HAMBURGER (1) ● ▲

8oz (230g) lean minced beef
1 small onion, very finely chopped
2 teaspoons water
Freshly ground black pepper

Preheat the grill to moderate. Mix all the ingredients well with your hands and shape into two balls. Flatten the balls between the palms of your hands and place on the grill rack. Grill for about 3 minutes on each side, or more, depending on how well done you like your meat. Season to taste. Serve hot or cold.

Calories per serving: 250   **Serves 2**

SLIMMER'S HAMBURGER (2)

8oz (230g) lean minced beef
1 medium egg
1oz (30g) onion, chopped
1 teaspoon mixed dried herbs
½ slice wholemeal bread, crumbed
Salt and pepper to taste

Place the meat, onion, herbs, salt and pepper in a bowl. Make a hole in the middle, break in the egg and mix well together. Shape the meat mixture into 2 balls and flatten them between the palms of your hands. Grill to taste, depending on how well done you like your meat.

Calories per serving: 280   **Serves 2**

BEEF AND VEGETABLE STEW ● ▲

8oz (230g) lean beef, cut into small cubes
2 large tomatoes, chopped
2 leeks, finely chopped
4oz (110g) button mushrooms
4fl.oz (110ml) water
Pepper
2 small bay leaves

Put all the ingredients into a saucepan and mix well. Stew over low heat for about 25 minutes, or until the beef is cooked and some of the liquid has evaporated to make the stew thicker.

Calories per serving: 220   **Serves 2**

BEEF GOULASH ● ▲

8oz (230g) lean beef, cut into small cubes
2 small bay leaves

Pepper
2 tablespoons paprika
½ pint (3dl) low-fat natural yogurt
2 medium-sized potatoes, peeled and cut into small cubes
2 small onions, very thinly sliced

Put all the ingredients into a saucepan and mix well.
Simmer over low heat, uncovered, for about 25 minutes, or
until the beef and potatoes are cooked and the stew has
thickened.

Calories per serving: 300   **Serves 2**

SPICED BEEF

8oz (230g) fillet steak, thinly sliced and cut into strips
2 tablespoons soy sauce
2 tablespoons lemon juice
3 tablespoons olive oil
1 green pepper, finely chopped
1 tablespoon finely chopped fresh ginger root
1 large garlic clove, chopped
8oz (230g) beansprouts, steamed

Put the steak in a small, shallow dish and pour the soy
sauce and lemon juice over it. Stir well to mix, and
marinate, stirring occasionally, for 1 hour. Drain the meat
and set it aside. Heat the oil in a small frying-pan and add
the pepper, ginger and garlic. Fry, stirring constantly, for
2 minutes. Add the beef and continue frying until it is
cooked. Put the beansprouts on a plate and add the meat.
Serve hot.

Calories per serving: 350   **Serve 2**

VEAL PIMIENTOS ● ▲

2 thin 4oz (110g) slices of veal
2oz (60g) onion, chopped
6oz (170g) green peppers, chopped
4oz (110g) button (or larger sliced) mushrooms
2½oz (75g) tomato purée, mixed with ½ pint (3dl) water
1 teaspoon mixed Italian seasoning; black pepper to taste

Place the onion, peppers and mushrooms on the veal
slices and roll into sausage shapes. Place in a baking dish
and cover with the diluted, seasoned purée. Bake at
425°F/220°C for about 40 minutes or until tender.

Calories per serving: 100   **Serves 2**

VEAL AND MUSHROOMS ● ▲

12oz (340g) veal fillet, cut into strips
4 small shallots, very finely sliced
4oz (110g) button mushrooms, halved

½ pint (3dl) low-fat natural yogurt
2 teaspoons paprika

Preheat the oven to 375°F/190°C. Mix all the ingredients except the paprika together and put them into a baking dish. Sprinkle over the paprika. Cover the dish with foil and bake for 25 minutes, or until the veal is tender. Serve hot.

Calories per serving: 270   **Serves 2**

CHICKEN CURRY ● ▲

6oz (170g) cooked chicken, diced (without skin)
4 tomatoes, chopped
4oz (110g) button mushrooms, halved
2 garlic cloves, crushed
1 teaspoon ground cumin
2 teaspoons garam masala
½ teaspoon chili powder
2 tablespoons water
4fl.oz (110ml) low-fat natural yogurt
8oz (230g) boiled beansprouts, hot (or tinned and heated)

Mix all the ingredients except the beansprouts together in a saucepan. Cover the pan and simmer for 20 minutes, stirring occasionally. Put the beansprouts on a warmed plate and pour over the curry. Serve immediately.

Calories per serving: 200   **Serves 2**

SPICED GRILLED CHICKEN ●

1 tablespoon soy sauce
2 teaspoons lemon juice
2 teaspoons prepared mustard
1 garlic clove, crushed
2 small chicken breasts (about 4oz/110g each)

Mix the soy sauce, lemon juice, mustard and garlic to a paste and spread them all over the chicken. Set aside in a cool place for 1 hour (this will allow the flavourings to seep into the meat). Preheat the grill to moderate. Line the grill rack with foil and place the chicken on it. Grill for about 7 minutes on each side, or until the chicken is cooked. Serve hot or cold.

Calories per serving: 260   **Serves 2**

STUFFED AUBERGINE OR MARROW ● ▲

2 aubergines or small marrows (3-4oz/90-110g)
8oz (230g) cold meat or chicken, chopped
1oz (30g) onion, chopped
1 garlic clove, crushed
2oz (60g) low-fat cheese, grated

1 tablespoon tomato purée

Cook aubergines or marrows gently until tender enough to scoop out without damaging skin. Cut in half and scoop out. Mix with all other ingredients except cheese and pile back in. Sprinkle with cheese and bake at 400°F/200°C for 25 minutes or until golden brown.
Calories per serving: 300 chicken, 400 meat Serves 2

"TARRAGON WINE" LIVER ▲

12oz (340g) calf's liver, thinly sliced
2oz (60g) onion, chopped
1 dessertspoon (10ml) red wine vinegar
Large sprig of parsley, chopped
1 teaspoon tarragon, chopped or dried
1oz (30g) low-fat spread
Black pepper to taste

Melt the low-fat spread in a medium saucepan. Add the onion and cook gently until tender. Add the liver and sauté for about 5 minutes. Then add the vinegar and tarragon, season with pepper and cook for a further 2 minutes. Serve hot, sprinkled with parsley.
Calories per serving: 370   **Serves 2**

COD IN PARSLEY SAUCE ● ▲

12oz (340g) cod steak
8oz (230g) boiled new potatoes, hot
½ pint (3dl) low-calorie white sauce, hot
(see Basic sauces, page 80)
2 tablespoons freshly chopped parsley

Poach the cod lightly in a little water. Drain and put on a heated plate. Surround with the potatoes. Mix the sauce with the parsley, pour over the fish and serve immediately.
Calories per serving: 370   **Serves 2**

COD ALMONDESA ▲

12oz (6oz/170g each) cod (or haddock) fillets
2 tablespoons parsley, chopped
2oz (60g) low-fat spread
2 tablespoons lemon juice
1oz (30g) almond flakes
½ fresh lemon

Place the fish in an ovenproof dish, pour the lemon juice over, dab the fat over the fish, and sprinkle with parsley and almond flakes. Bake at 400°F/200°C for about 25 minutes. Serve with a ¼ lemon wedge on the side.
Calories per serving: 320   **Serves 2**

Salads

CHICKEN SALAD ●▲

4fl.oz (110ml) low-fat natural yogurt
2 teaspoons lemon juice
Pepper
8oz (230g) cooked chicken, cut into strips
2 bunches mustard and cress

Mix the yogurt, lemon juice and pepper together. Put all the remaining ingredients in a bowl, pour the yogurt dressing over, toss well and serve.

Calories per serving: 200 **Serves 2**

CURRIED CHICKEN MAYONNAISE ●▲

3 tablespoons low-calorie mayonnaise
1 tablespoon lemon juice
1 tablespoon curry powder
12oz (340g) cooked chicken meat, cut into strips
4 large lettuce leaves
4 medium tomatoes, sliced

Mix the mayonnaise, lemon juice and curry powder together in a bowl. Add the chicken and stir well to mix. Line a plate with the lettuce leaves and pile the chicken mixture in the middle. Arrange the sliced tomatoes around the edge of the plate and serve.

Calories per serving: 300 **Serves 2**

SALMON SALAD ▲

4 large lettuce leaves
12oz (340g) salmon steak, poached in a little water
with 1 tablespoon vinegar or lemon juice
8 large radishes, sliced
4 tomatoes, sliced
8 spring onions
1 lemon, cut into wedges

Lay the lettuce leaves on a plate and put the salmon steak on top. Arrange the salad vegetables and lemon wedges decoratively around the salmon, and serve.

Calories per serving: 360 **Serves 2**

COLESLAW SALAD ●▲

2 tablespoons low-calorie salad cream
¼ teaspoon prepared mustard
Pepper
4oz (110g) white cabbage, coarsely shredded
2 medium carrots, shredded

1 small onion, very thinly sliced

Mix the salad dressing, mustard and pepper together and add the vegetables. Toss well, chill and serve.

Calories per serving: 50　　　　　　　　　　**Serves 2**

CARROT, APPLE AND NUT SALAD ▲

12oz (340g) raw carrot, peeled and grated
1oz (30g) fresh peanuts
2 small eating apples, cored and diced
2 teaspoons lemon juice
1 tablespoon cider vinegar
Pepper

Mix all the ingredients together, chill and serve.

Calories per serving: 150　　　　　　　　　　**Serves 2**

ENDIVE SALAD ▲

2 teaspoons olive oil
1 tablespoon tarragon vinegar
Pepper
½ teaspoon prepared mustard
1 small curly endive, chopped
2oz (60g) small mushrooms, thinly sliced
½oz (15g) peanuts, chopped

Mix the olive oil, vinegar, pepper and mustard together. Put all the vegetables and nuts in a salad bowl, pour over the dressing, toss well and serve.

Calories per serving: 80　　　　　　　　　　**Serves 2**

ENDIVE AND WALNUT SALAD ▲

½ small curly endive, coarsely chopped
1oz (30g) chopped walnuts
2oz (60g) raw button mushrooms, thinly sliced
1 tablespoon olive oil
2 teaspoons lemon juice
1 tablespoon vinegar
2 teaspoons French mustard
1 garlic clove, crushed; pepper

Put the endive, walnuts and mushrooms into a salad bowl. Mix the remaining dressing ingredients together and pour them over the salad. Toss well and serve.

Calories per serving: 130　　　　　　　　　　**Serves 2**

CHEESE, ORANGE AND WATERCRESS SALAD

4 tablespoons low-fat natural yogurt
2 tablespoons lemon juice

Pepper
2 bunches watercress, chopped
2 large oranges, peeled and chopped
4oz (110g) Edam cheese, chopped

Mix the yogurt, lemon juice, salt and pepper together in a small salad bowl. Add the remaining ingredients, toss well and serve.

Calories per serving: 200   **Serves 2**

CHICORY, ORANGE AND WATERCRESS SALAD ●▲

2 heads chicory, thinly sliced
2 oranges, peeled, halved and thinly sliced
2 bunches watercress, chopped
1 tablespoon tarragon vinegar
2 teaspoons lemon juice
1 teaspoon French mustard
Pepper

Put the chicory, orange and watercress into a salad bowl. Mix the remaining ingredients together and pour them over the salad. Toss well and serve.

Calories per serving: 60   **Serves 2**

Basic sauces

LOW-CALORIE WHITE SAUCE

½ pint (3dl) skimmed milk
1oz (30g) plain flour
½oz (15g) margarine

Melt the fat in a saucepan, add the flour and cook for a few minutes, stirring constantly. Then slowly add the milk, stirring slowly, and cook over a low heat until the sauce thickens.

Calories per fl.oz: 40

May be used to make savoury sauces by adding tomato purée, meat stock, low-fat cheese, etc.

LOW-CALORIE ONION SAUCE

½ pint (3dl) skimmed milk
1oz (30g) plain flour
1oz (30g) margarine
7oz (200g) onion, chopped and boiled
¼ teaspoon salt; pepper to taste

Make white sauce as above, adding the onion when the

sauce is cooked to the correct smoothness, and stir well.
Calories per fl. oz: 25

Desserts and cakes

FRUIT CREAM ●▲■

2oz (60g) dried skimmed milk
4oz (110g) fruit (strawberries, raspberries, black
currants or cooked apples), fresh or frozen
½oz (15g) gelatin
½ pint (3dl) water, warmed
Liquid sweetener to taste

Melt the gelatin in the warmed water. Mash the fruit in a
blender, add milk and sweetener, and whip the mixture
until it is creamy in texture.
Calories per fl. oz: 15   **Serves 2**

GOOSEBERRY FOOL ●▲■

1lb (450g) dessert gooseberries
2 tablespoons water
½ pint (3dl) low-fat natural yogurt
Liquid sweetener to taste

Put the gooseberries and water into a saucepan and cover
the pan. Cook over low heat until the gooseberries are
quite mushy. Remove the pan from the heat and mash the
gooseberries with a fork until they form a purée. Stir in the
yogurt and enough sweetener to taste. Chill before
serving.
Calories per serving: 160   **Serves 2**

PLUM COMPOTE ●▲■

1lb (450g) ripe dessert plums, halved and stoned
Grated rind of 1 lemon
Pinch of allspice
4 tablespoons water

Put all the ingredients in a saucepan and cover the pan.
Cook over gentle heat until the plums are very tender and
beginning to go mushy. Chill and serve.
Calories per serving: 80   **Serves 2**

APPLE AND ORANGE COMPOTE ●▲■

4 medium cooking apples, peeled, cored and sliced
2oz (60g) sultanas
Juice and grated rind of 1 large orange

Liquid sweetener to taste

Put the apples, sultanas, orange rind and juice into a saucepan. Cover the pan and simmer until the apples are tender and beginning to disintegrate. Remove the pan from the heat and add sweetener to taste. Serve chilled.

Calories per serving: 140   **Serves 2**

FRUIT "ICE" ●▲■

5oz (140g) low-fat natural yogurt
½oz (15g) gelatin
1 teaspoon lemon juice
4oz (110g) fruit (strawberries, raspberries, black currants or cooked apples), fresh or frozen
Liquid sweetener to taste

Melt the gelatin in 2 tablespoons warm water, and add the lemon juice and yogurt. Mash the fruit in a blender, add the sweetener, then blend in the gelatin-and-yogurt mix until the consistency is fluffy. Chill and serve.

Calories per serving: 75   **Serves 2**

ICED MELON MOUSSE ●▲■

12oz (340g) wedge of honeydew melon
1 teaspoon ground ginger
Liquid sweetener to taste
4 egg whites, stiffly whipped

Scoop the flesh out of the melon and blend it in a blender, or rub it through a strainer. Put the puréed melon into a bowl and stir in the ginger, with enough liquid sweetener to taste. Fold in the egg whites and pour the mixture into a small dish. Chill for 2 hours before serving.

Calories per serving: 50   **Serves 2**

RASPBERRY CREAM ●▲■

8oz (230g) fresh raspberries
½ pint (3dl) low-fat yogurt
Liquid sweetener to taste

Mash the raspberries with a fork and stir them into the yogurt. Add enough sweetener to taste. Serve chilled.

Calories per serving: 60

APRICOT MOUSSE ●▲■

3oz (90g) dried apricot halves
½ pint (3dl) water
4 strips lemon rind
8fl.oz (230ml) low-fat natural yogurt

2 large egg whites, stiffly whipped

Soak the apricots in the water for 2 hours. Put the apricots and water in a saucepan with the lemon rind, and simmer until the apricots are very tender and beginning to turn mushy. Rub the mixture through a strainer and let it cool. Stir in the yogurt and then fold in the egg whites. Chill before serving.

Calories per serving: 150　　　　　　　　　**Serves 2**

PRUNE WHIP ●▲■

4oz (110g) dried stoned prunes
½ pint (3dl) water
4 strips orange rind
½ pint (3dl) low-fat natural yogurt

Soak the prunes in the water for 2 hours. Put the prunes and water into a saucepan with the orange rind. Cover the pan and simmer until the prunes are very tender and beginning to go mushy. Rub them through a strainer. Using a fork, beat in the yogurt. Chill before serving.

Calories per serving: 160　　　　　　　　　**Serves 2**

APPLE SNOW ●▲■

8oz (230g) sweet eating apples, peeled and cored
Grated orange or lemon rind
2 tablespoons water
1 large egg white, stiffly beaten

Slice the apples thinly and put them in a saucepan with the rind and water. Cover the pan and cook gently, stirring occasionally, until the apples are soft. Rub the apples through a strainer and let them cool. Fold in the egg white and chill before serving.

Calories per serving: 90　　　　　　　　　**Serves 2**

EGG CUSTARD ▲■

7fl.oz (200ml) low-fat milk
2 eggs (small)
Liquid sweetener to taste
2 drops vanilla extract (optional)

Mix all the ingredients together thoroughly in a small heat-proof bowl. Set the bowl over a pan of barely simmering water and cook, stirring constantly, until the custard is thick enough to coat the back of the spoon. Pour into a small dish. Serve hot or cold.

This can be flavoured with strong black coffee or cocoa powder to make coffee cream or chocolate cream.

Calories per serving: 125
Makes about 9fl.oz (260ml).　　　　　　　**Serves 2**

LOW-CALORIE CUSTARD ● ▲ ■

$\frac{1}{2}$ pint (3dl) low-fat milk
2 drops vanilla extract
2 teaspoons cornflour, mixed with 1 tablespoon water
Liquid sweetener to taste

Put the milk, vanilla extract and cornflour into a small saucepan and cook over moderate heat, stirring, until the custard has thickened. Remove the pan from the heat and stir in sweetener to taste. Serve hot or cold.

Calories per serving: 80   **Serves 2**

SCOTCH PANCAKES

8oz (230g) self-raising flour
1 tablespoon sugar
2 eggs
Approx $\frac{1}{3}$ pint (2dl) milk
Pinch of salt

Place dry ingredients in a bowl and add eggs. Beat, gradually adding milk, until a fairly stiff batter is achieved. Either fry in *very shallow* corn oil or cook on a griddle.

Calories each: 45   **Makes 25**

DROP SCONES ● ▲ ■

7oz (200g) plain flour
1$\frac{1}{2}$oz (45g) margarine
$\frac{1}{3}$ pint (200ml) skimmed milk
1 egg
$\frac{1}{2}$oz (15g) caster sugar
Pinch (less than $\frac{1}{4}$ teaspoon) salt
$\frac{1}{2}$ level teaspoon baking powder (bicarbonate of soda)
1 level teaspoon cream of tartar

Sift the flour with the baking powder and cream of tartar, rub in the fat and mix in the caster sugar. Stir in the milk and egg, and beat to a stiff batter. Drop the batter by the teaspoonful onto a hot griddle greased with not more than $\frac{1}{2}$oz (15g) of margarine.

Calories each: 40   **Makes about 30**
                                        $\frac{1}{2}$oz (15g) scones

Food composition and Calorie tables

Tables 1 and 2 in this section answer the often-asked question: Is such-and-such a good food? There is no *yes* or *no* answer because almost all foods supply some nutrients. The answer depends on: (1) how much of the nutrient or nutrients is present in a standard amount of the food, and (2) how much of that food is eaten.

Different samples of the same food can differ considerably in their nutrient content. Meat, for example, can vary from sample to sample in the amount of fat, of water, and therefore of protein; and there is even greater variation in the amounts of mineral salts and particularly of vitamins in different samples of the same food. To avoid giving a false impression of precise figures, foods are listed in tables 1 and 2 as "useful" (△) or "rich" (▲) sources of nutrients, except in regard to their energy and carbohydrate content, where figures are quoted.

HOW TO USE TABLE 1

A food is considered to be a "useful" source if it contains **10 percent** of the recommended daily amount (RDA) in 100 grams and as a "rich" source if it contains **25 percent** or more of the RDA.

Symbol:	10% RDA △	25% RDA ▲
Protein (g)	7	18
Calcium (mg)	50	125
Iron (mg)	1	2.5
Vitamin A (µg)	75	200
Vitamin C (mg)	3	8
Riboflavin (mg)	0.17	0.4
Thiamin (mg)	0.12	0.3
Niacin (mg)	1.8	5

Such a method of judging a food as "useful" or "rich" is arbitrary but may be helpful.

Energy is quoted in kilojoules and kilocalories per 100g, but this, again, varies with the particular sample of food and is useful as a guide rather than being a precise figure—as is the carbohydrate content, which is quoted in grams per 100g of food.

Fats Since an excessive intake of fats is thought to be potentially harmful, foods supplying more than **20 percent** of their total calories as fat are marked ○ and those supplying more than **40 percent** are marked ●.

HOW TO USE TABLE 2

Foods that are a "useful" source of nutrients according to Table 1 may be eaten in such small amounts that they contribute little to the diet. Conversely, if large amounts are eaten "useful" sources may make a major contribution. So table 2 takes into account the amount of food eaten, although actual portions will obviously vary a great deal from the suggested average.

Since a portion of food may amount to a whole dish the standards have been changed; in table 2 a portion of food is considered to make a "useful" (△) contribution to the whole diet if it supplies **one-sixth** of the RDA of the nutrient, and "rich" (▲) if it contributes **half** the RDA.

	one-sixth RDA	half RDA
Symbol:	△	▲
Protein (g)	12	35
Calcium (mg)	80	250
Iron (mg)	2	5
Vitamin A (μg)	125	375
Vitamin C (mg)	5	15
Riboflavin (mg)	0.3	0.8
Thiamin (mg)	0.2	0.6
Niacin (mg)	3	9

Fats As in table 1, foods providing more than **20 percent** of their total calories as fat are marked ○ and those providing more than **40 percent** are marked ●.

Notes (1) Portions marked * are from the recipes in this book on pages 67–84.

(2) Table 3 (pages 124–6) provides figures for dietary fibre per 100g for a wide variety of foods.

KEY TO TABLE 1
△ = 10% RDA
▲ = 25% RDA
○ = 20+ % fat
● = 40+ % fat

Table 1
Nutritional values per 100 g

	Kilojoules	Kilocalories	Carbohydrate	Protein	Calcium	Iron	Vitamin A	Vitamin C	Riboflavin	Thiamin	Niacin	Fat
Ackee, canned	600	140	0					▲				●
Advocaat, liqueur	1100	260	28									
Ale, *see* Beer												
All-Bran (Kellogg's)	1050	250	46	△	△	▲			▲	▲	▲	
Almonds	2500	600	5	▲	▲	▲			▲	△	△	●
Anchovies, canned, drained	1200	290	0	▲	▲	▲					△	●
Apple crumble	900	200	37									○
Apples	150	35	10									
baked without sugar	165	40	10									
stewed with sugar	280	65	18									
without sugar	150	35	10									
Apricots, canned with sugar syrup	450	110	30				▲					
Apricots, raw	120	30	7				▲	△				
weighed with stones	100	25	6				▲	△				
Apricots, dried	800	190	45				▲		△	△		
stewed with sugar	350	80	20				▲					
without sugar	300	70	16				▲					
Apricots, stewed with sugar (without stones)	260	60	16				▲	△				
(with stones)	240	55	15				▲	△				
Apricots, stewed without sugar (without stones)	100	25	6				▲	△				
(with stones)	90	20	5				▲	△				
Arrowroot	1500	360	94									
Artichoke, globe, boiled (50% waste)	30	7	0					△				
Artichoke, Jerusalem, boiled	80	20	0									
Aubergine, raw	60	15	0					△				
Aubergine, stuffed with chicken*	630	150	0	▲	▲		△	△			▲	●
Avocado pear	900	210	0		△		▲					●
Bacon, collar joint, boiled	1350	330	0	▲		△			△	▲	△	●
lean only	800	200	0	▲		△			△	▲	△	●
Bacon, fried, back	1900	460	0	▲		△			△	▲	▲	●
middle	2000	480	0	▲		△			△	▲	▲	●
streaky	2000	480	0	▲		△			△	▲	▲	●
Bacon, gammon joint, boiled	1110	270	0	▲		△			△	▲	△	●
lean only	700	170	0	▲		△			△	▲	▲	○
Bacon, grilled, back	1700	400	0	▲		△			△	▲	▲	●
middle	1700	400	0	▲		△			△	▲	▲	●
streaky	1750	420	0	▲		△			△	▲	▲	●
Bamboo shoots, canned	100	25	4									
Banana	350	85	20					▲				
Barcelona nuts	2700	650	5	△	▲	▲			△	△	△	●
Barley, pearl, cooked	500	120	28									
Barley, pearl, raw	1540	360	84	△							△	○
Barley, whole grain, raw	1400	330	69	△	△	▲				▲	▲	

Table 1
(per 100 g)
continued

Be-Bi

	Kilojoules	Kilocalories	Carbohydrate	Protein	Calcium	Iron	Vitamin A	Vitamin C	Riboflavin	Thiamin	Niacin	Fat
boiled	470	110	23			△					△	
Beans, broad, boiled	200	50	7			△		▲			△	
Beans, butter, boiled	400	100	17	△		△				▲	△	
Beans, French, boiled	30	7	0				△	△				
Beans, haricot, boiled	400	100	17		△	▲				▲	△	
canned in tomato sauce	270	60	10			△						
Beans, mung, raw	1000	240	36	▲	△	▲			△	▲	△	
cooked	450	100	11			△						
Beans, runner, boiled	80	20	0				△	△				
Beans, valor, canned	80	20	3									
Beansprouts, canned	40	10	0		△							
Beef, corned, canned	900	210	0	▲		▲			△		△	●
Beef, forerib, roast	1500	360	0	▲		△			△		△	●
Beef, rump steak, fried	1000	240	0	▲		▲			△		▲	●
grilled	900	220	0	▲		▲			△		▲	●
Beef, silverside, boiled	1000	240	0	▲		▲			△		△	●
lean only	750	180	0	▲		▲			△		△	○
Beef, sirloin, roast	1200	290	0	▲		△			△		▲	●
lean only	800	190	0	▲		△			△		▲	●
Beef, spiced *	550	130	0	△		▲		▲			△	●
Beef, stewing steak	900	210	0	▲		△			△		△	●
Beef, topside, roast	900	210	0		▲		▲				△	△	●
lean only	650	150	0		▲		▲				△	△	●
Beef brisket, boiled	1350	330	0	▲		▲			△		▲	●
Beefburger, fried	1100	260	7	▲		▲			△		▲	●
Beef goulash*	420	100	6	△	△				△			○
Beef mince, stewed	1000	240	0	▲		▲			△		△	●
Beef-stuffed aubergine*	780	190	0	▲	▲	△			△		△	●
Beef and vegetable stew *	380	90	2	△	·	△		△	△		△	●
Beer, ale, pale bottled	135	32	2									
strong	300	70	6									
Beer, bitter, draught	130	30	2									
Beer, bitter, keg	130	30	2									
Beer, brown ale	120	30	3									
Beer, canned bitter	130	30	2									
Beer, lager, bottled or canned	120	30	1·5									
Beer, mild, draught	100	25	2									
Beer, stout, bottled	155	37	4									
extra stout	163	40	2									
Beetroot, boiled	190	45	10					△				
Bemax	1500	350	45	▲		▲			▲	▲	▲	○
Bengal gram (dahl), cooked	600	140	22	△	△	▲	△			△		
Bilberries, raw	250	60	15					▲				
Biscuit, chocolate	2200	520	67		△	△						●

Table 1

Bi-Ca

Key △ = 10% RDA
▲ = 25% RDA
○ = 20+ % fat
● = 40+ % fat

	Kilojoules	Kilocalories	Carbohydrate	Protein	Calcium	Iron	Vitamin A	Vitamin C	Riboflavin	Thiamin	Niacin	Fat
Biscuit, cream cracker	1860	440	68	△	△	△				△		○
Biscuit, custard cream	2150	510	69		△	△				△		●
Biscuit, digestive, chocolate-coated	2100	490	67	△	△	△						●
Biscuit, digestive, plain	2000	480	66	△	△	△				△		●
Biscuit, ginger nut	1900	450	79		▲	▲						○
Biscuit, plain (semi-sweet)	1900	450	75	△	▲	△				△	△	○
Biscuit, wafer (cream-filled)	2200	530	66		△	△						●
Biscuit, water	1850	440	76	△	▲	△						○
Blackberries, raw	125	30	6		△	△		▲				
stewed without sugar	100	25	6		△			▲				
with sugar	250	60	15		△			▲				
Bloater, grilled	1000	240	0	▲	▲	▲			△		△	●
weighed with bones	800	190	0	▲	△	△					△	●
Brain, calf, boiled	650	150	0	△		△			△		△	●
Brain, lamb, boiled	500	120	0	△		△			△		△	●
Bran, wheat	880	200	27	△	△	▲			▲	▲	▲	○
Bran Buds (Kellogg's) (wheat)	1070	250	50	△	△	▲			▲	▲	▲	
Brandy	920	220	0									
Bran Flakes (Kellogg's) (wheat)	1320	320	68	△	△	▲			▲	▲	▲	
Brawn	600	150	0	△		△						
Brazil nuts	2500	600	5	△	▲	▲				▲		●
Bread, brown	950	220	45	△	△	▲				△	△	
Hovis	970	230	45	△	▲	▲				▲	△	
white	990	230	50	△	△	△				△		
white, toasted	1270	300	65	△	△	△				△	△	
dried, crumbs	1500	350	78	△	▲	▲				△	△	
wholemeal	920	220	42	△	△	▲				△	△	
Bread, West Indian	1200	280	59	△	▲	▲				△		
Bread-and-butter pudding	700	170	17		▲		△		△			●
Breakfast cereals, *see* separate entries												
Broccoli, tops, boiled	80	20	0		△	△	▲	▲	△			
Brussels sprouts, raw	100	25	0			△		▲				
boiled	75	20	0			△		▲				
Buns, currant	1300	300	55	△	△	▲						○
Butter	3000	740	0				▲					●
Cabbage, red, raw	85	20	0		△			▲				
Cabbage, Savoy, raw	100	25	0		△		△	▲				
boiled	40	10	0		△		△	▲				
Cabbage, spring, boiled	30	7	0				△	▲				
Cabbage, white, raw	90	20	0					▲				
Cabbage, winter, raw	90	20	0		△			▲				
boiled	70	15	0					▲				
Cake, Chinese rice flour	1200	300	60			△						
Cake, fancy, iced	1700	400	70			△						○

Table 1
(per 100 g)
continued   Ca-Ch

	Kilojoules	Kilocalories	Carbohydrate	Protein	Calcium	Iron	Vitamin A	Vitamin C	Riboflavin	Thiamin	Niacin	Fat
Cake, fruit	1400	330	60		△	△						●
Cake, ginger bread	1570	370	63	▲	▲	△						○
Cake, Madeira	1650	390	58		△							●
Cake, rock	1660	400	60	▲	△	△						●
Cake, sponge, with fat	1950	460	53	▲	△	▲						●
without fat	1300	300	54	△	△	△			△	△		○
jam-filled	1300	300	64	△	△	△						
Carrot, old, raw	100	25	5		△		▲	△				
boiled	80	20	4				▲	△				
canned	80	20	4				▲	△				
Carrot, young, boiled	90	20	4				▲	△				
Cauliflower, raw	60	10	0					▲				
boiled	40	10	0					▲				
Cauliflower cheese *	250	60	5	▲				▲	△			●
Celeriac, boiled	40	10	0	△								
Celery, raw	40	10	0		△			△				
boiled	20	5	0		△			△				
Celery soup *	90	22	3	△								
Chapatis, made with fat	1420	340	50	△	△	▲				△	△	○
without fat	860	200	44	△	△	▲				△	△	
Cheese, Camembert	1250	300	0	▲	▲		▲		▲			●
Cheddar	1700	410	0	▲	▲		▲		▲			●
cottage	400	100	1	△	△				△			
cream	1800	440	0		△				△			●
Danish blue	1470	360	0	▲	▲		▲		▲			●
Edam	1260	300	0	▲	▲		▲		▲			●
feta	1000	240	0	△	▲		△		△			●
Parmesan	1700	410	0	▲	▲		▲		▲			●
processed	1300	310	0	▲	▲		▲		△			●
spread	1200	290	1	▲	▲		▲		△			●
Stilton	1920	460	0	▲	▲		▲		△			●
Cheese, cauliflower *	250	60	5	▲				▲	△			●
Cheese, macaroni *	525	125	14	△	▲							●
Cheesecake	1800	430	25	△	△	▲						●
Cherries, glacé	900	210	56		△	▲						
Cherries, raw, with stones	175	40	10					△				
without stones	200	50	12					△				
Cherries, stewed, with sugar, weighed with stones	300	70	18									
without stones	330	80	20									
Cherries, stewed without sugar, with stones	140	35	8									
weighed without stones	170	40	10									
Cherry brandy	1100	260	33									
Chestnuts	700	170	37						△	△		

Table 1

Key
△ = 10% RDA
▲ = 25% RDA
○ = 20+ % fat
● = 40+ % fat

	Kilojoules	Kilocalories	Carbohydrate	Protein	Calcium	Iron	Vitamin A	Vitamin C	Riboflavin	Thiamin	Niacin	Fat
Chicken, boiled	770	180	0	▲		△			△		▲	●
white meat	700	160	0	▲							▲	○
dark meat	850	200	0	▲		△			△		▲	●
Chicken, roast, with skin	900	210	0	▲					△		▲	●
meat only	620	150	0	▲					△		▲	
light meat	600	140	0	▲							▲	
dark meat	650	160	0	▲		△			△		▲	
Chicken, spiced and grilled *	970	230	0	▲							△	●
Chicken, wing (meat only— weighed with bone)	300	70	0	△							△	○
leg (meat only— weighed with bone)	400	100	0	△							▲	○
Chicken curry *	300	70	2	△							△	○
Chicken-liver pâté *	400	95	2	▲		▲	▲	▲	△	△	△	●
Chicken omelet *	760	180	0	▲			△	△	▲		△	●
Chicken-stuffed aubergine*	630	150	0	▲	▲				△	△	▲	
Chickpeas, cooked	600	140	22	△	△	▲	△			△		
Chicory, raw	40	10	0					△				
Chocolate, *Bounty* bar	2000	470	58		△	△						●
Chocolate, *Mars* bar	1850	440	67	▲	△				△			●
Chocolate, plain	2200	530	65			△						●
milk	2200	530	60	△	▲	△			△			●
Chocolates, filled	1900	450	75		△	△						●
Chutney, apple	800	190	50									
tomato	660	160	40		△		△	△				
Cider, dry	150	36	3									
sweet	180	40	4									
vintage	420	100	7									
Clementines, *see* Tangerines												
Cobnuts	1500	360	7	△		△				▲		●
Coca-Cola	170	40	11									
Cockles, boiled, without shells	200	50	0	△	▲	▲						
Cocoa powder	1300	310	12	▲	▲	▲				△	△	●
Coco Krispies (Kellogg's) (rice)	1490	360	87			▲			▲	▲	▲	
Coconut	1500	360	4			△						●
desiccated	2500	600	6			▲						●
Coconut milk	90	20	5									
Cod, dried, salted	600	140	0	▲		△						
Cod, smoked raw	350	80	0	▲								
poached	430	100	0	▲								
Cod almondesa *	670	160	0	△	△	△	△	△	△	△		●
Cod fillet, baked	400	100	0	▲								
weighed with bones and skin	350	80	0	▲								
Cod fillet, fried	750	180	0	▲								●
in batter	850	200	10	▲								●

Table 1
(per 100 g)
continued

Co-Da

	Kilojoules	Kilocalories	Carbohydrate	Protein	Calcium	Iron	Vitamin A	Vitamin C	Riboflavin	Thiamin	Niacin	Fat
Cod fillet, grilled	400	100	0	▲								
Cod fillet, poached	400	100	0	▲								
weighed with bones and skin	350	80	0	▲								
Cod fillet, steamed	350	80	0	▲								
weighed with bones and skin	300	70	0	▲								
Cod in parsley sauce •	390	90	11	△	△			△				
Cod-liver oil	3700	900	0				▲					●
Consommé with vegetables •	70	16	5			▲	▲					
Corn Flakes (Kellogg's)	1440	340	82	△		▲			▲	▲	▲	
Corn-on-the-cob, boiled	520	120	23			△	△			△	△	
Cornflour	1500	350	92			△						
Cornish pastie	1400	330	30	△	△	△						●
Cornmeal, unsifted, uncooked	1500	350	72	△		△				△		
sifted	1550	370	73	△		△				△		
Cottonseed oil	3700	900	0									●
Country Store (Kellogg's)	1480	350	68	△	▲	▲			▲	▲	▲	
Courgettes, raw	100	25	5			△	△	▲				
Couscous (millet)	950	230	51			▲				△		
Crab, boiled	550	130	0	▲		△			△	△	△	○
weighed with shell	100	25	0									○
Crab, canned	340	80	0	▲	▲	▲						
Cranberries, cooked, sweetened	750	180	45									
Cranberries, raw	60	15	0			△		▲				
Cranberry sauce, sweetened	750	180	45									
Cream, canned, sterilized (23% fat)	950	230	3		△		▲					●
double (48% fat)	1850	450	2		△		▲					●
single (20% fat)	880	210	3		△		▲					●
whipping (35% fat)	1350	330	3		△		▲					●
Crispbread, rye	1370	320	71	△	△	▲				▲		
Crispbread, wheat, starch-reduced	1640	390	37	▲	△	▲				△	△	
Crisps, potato	2200	530	50			△		▲		△	△	●
Cucumber, raw	40	10	0					△				
Crunchy Nut Cornflakes (Kellogg's)	1550	370	79	△		▲			▲	▲	▲	
Curaçao	1300	310	28									
Custard, egg •	360	85	4	△	△				△			●
Custard, egg, baked	500	120	11	▲		△			△			●
Custard, low-calorie •	210	50	8	▲					△			
Custard (from powder)	500	120	17	▲					△			○
Custard powder	1500	350	92	△								
Dahl (Bengal gram), cooked	600	140	22	△	△	▲	△			△		
Dahl, cooked (from Mung beans)	450	100	11			▲	△					○
Dahl, masur (from lentils)	400	100	11			△						○
Damsons, raw, with stones	150	35	10									

Table 1   Da-Fr

Key △ = 10% RDA ▲ = 25% RDA ○ = 20+ % fat ● = 40+ % fat

	Kilojoules	Kilocalories	Carbohydrate	Protein	Calcium	Iron	Vitamin A	Vitamin C	Riboflavin	Thiamin	Niacin	Fat
without stones	160	38	10									
Damsons, stewed with sugar, weighed with stones	270	65	17									
weighed without stones	290	70	18									
Damsons, stewed without sugar, weighed with stones	130	30	7									
weighed without stones	140	33	8									
Dates, dried, with stones	900	210	55		△	△					△	
without stones	1000	240	65		△	△					△	
Dogfish, fried in batter	1100	260	8	△		▲					△	○
weighed with skin and bone	1000	240	7	△		▲					△	○
Doughnuts	1500	360	50		△	△						●
Dripping	3700	900	0									●
Duck, roast	1400	330	0	▲		▲			▲	▲	▲	●
meat only	800	190	0	▲		▲			▲	▲	▲	●
Dumpling (flour-suet)	900	220	25		▲							●
Éclairs, chocolate, cream-filled	1570	380	38		△	△	▲					●
Eel, stewed	700	180	0	△			▲		△	△	△	●
Egg custard *	360	85	4	△	△				△			
Eggs, whole	610	150	0	△	△	△	△		▲			
whole, dried	2300	560	0	▲	▲	△	△		▲	▲		
white	150	35	0	△					▲			
yolk	1400	340	0	△	▲	△	△		▲	▲		●
Egg, duck	800	200	0	△	△	▲	△		▲	△		
Egg, scrambled, with asparagus *	420	100	0		△	△	△	△				●
Egg, scrambled, with smoked salmon *	710	170	0	▲		△	△		▲	△		●
Endive, raw	50	12	0			▲	▲	▲				
Extra (Kellogg's)	1380	330	60	△	▲	▲			▲	▲	▲	
Faggots	1000	240	15	△	△	▲	▲		▲	△	△	●
Fat, cooking	3700	900	0									●
Figs, dried	900	210	50		▲	▲						
stewed without sugar	500	120	30		▲	▲						
Figs, fresh	175	40	10									
Fish cakes, frozen	500	120	17	△	△	△						
fried	800	200	15	△	△	△						●
Fish fingers, frozen	750	180	16	△								○
fried	1000	240	17	△								●
Fish paste	700	170	4	△	▲	▲			△		△	●
Fish pie, with potato and milk	500	120	12	△								○
Flour, chapati, white	1400	330	77	△	△	△				△	△	
brown, coarse	1400	330	73	△	△	△				△	△	
Flour, white	1400	340	75	△	▲	△				▲	△	
Flour, wholemeal	1350	320	66	△						▲	▲	
Frankfurters	1100	260	3	△	.	△						●
French dressing	2700	660	0									●

Table 1
(per 100 g)
continued

Fr-Ha

	Kilojoules	Kilocalories	Carbohydrate	Protein	Calcium	Iron	Vitamin A	Vitamin C	Riboflavin	Thiamin	Niacin	Fat
Frosties (Kellogg's) (maize)	1470	350	88			▲			▲	▲	▲	
Fruit pie filling, canned	400	95	25									
Fruit salad, canned in syrup	400	95	25									
Gari, raw (fermented cassava)	1450	350	83			△						
Ghee, butter	3600	860	0				▲					●
vegetable	3600	860	0									●
Gin	920	220	0									
Golden syrup	1270	300	79									
Goose, roast	1300	310	0	▲		▲			▲	▲	▲	●
Gooseberries, dessert	150	35	10					▲				
Gooseberries, green, raw	70	17	0					▲				
stewed without sugar	60	14	0					▲				
with sugar	200	50	12					▲				
Goulash, beef *	420	100	6	△	△				△			○
Granadilla, pulp only	150	35	6			△		▲				
weighed whole	60	15	3					▲				
Grapefruit, flesh only	100	25	5					▲				
whole fruit	50	12	3					▲				
canned in syrup	250	60	16					▲				
Grapefruit juice, unsweetened	130	30	8					▲				
sweetened	165	40	10					▲				
Grapefruit peel, candied	1350	320	80									
Grape juice	270	65	17									
Grapenuts (General Foods)	1500	350	76	△		▲	▲		▲	▲	▲	
Grapes, with skin and pips	220	50	13					△				
flesh only	260	60	16					△				
Greengages, raw, with stones	190	45	11									
without stones	200	50	12									
Greengages, stewed with sugar, with stones	300	70	20									
without stones	320	75	20									
Greengages, stewed without sugar, with stones	160	38	10									
without stones	170	40	11									
Ground-nut oil	3700	900	0									●
Grouse, roast, with bone	500	120	0	▲		▲			▲	△	▲	○
without bone	700	170	0	▲		▲			▲	▲	▲	○
Guava, whole, raw	250	60	15					▲				
Guava, canned in syrup	260	60	16					▲				
Gums, fruit	750	180	45									
Haddock, fried	700	170	0	▲	△	△					△	●
weighed with bones	650	150	0	▲	△	△					△	●
Haddock, smoked, steamed	430	100	0	▲	△	△					△	
weighed with skin and bones	280	65	0	△							△	
Haddock, steamed	420	100	0	▲	△						△	

Table 1

Key △ = 10% RDA ▲ = 25% RDA ○ = 20+% fat ● = 40+% fat

	Kilojoules	Kilocalories	Carbohydrate	Protein	Calcium	Iron	Vitamin A	Vitamin C	Riboflavin	Thiamin	Niacin	Fat
weighed with bones	320	75	0	▲							△	
Haggis	1300	300	20	△		▲	▲		△	△		●
Halibut, steamed	550	130	0	▲							▲	○
weighed with skin and bones	400	100	0	▲							△	○
Halva (Greek)	2500	600	54	△	△	▲				▲	△	●
Halwa (Indian)	1650	400	27	△	△	▲			▲	▲	▲	●
Ham, canned	500	120	0	▲		△			△	▲	△	○
Ham and pork, chopped, canned	1100	260	0	△		△			△	△	▲	●
Hamburger, dieter's (1) •	840	200	0	△		▲			△		△	●
Hamburger, dieter's (2) •	760	180	2	△		△			△		△	●
Hare, stewed (weighed with bones)	600	140	0	▲		▲			△		▲	●
meat	800	200	0	▲		▲			△		▲	●
Hazelnuts	1500	360	7	△		△				▲		●
Heart, ox, stewed	750	180	0	▲		▲		▲	▲	▲	▲	●
Heart, sheep, roast	1000	240	0	▲		▲		▲	▲	▲	▲	●
Herring, fried	1000	240	0	▲		△			△		△	●
weighed with bones	850	200	0	▲		△			△		△	●
Hominy grits, raw (maize)	1500	360	78	△		△	△			△		
Honey	1200	290	76									
Honeycomb	1200	290	76									
Horseradish, raw	250	60	0		▲	△		▲				
Huevos flamencos •	270	65	3	△	△	▲			△			●
Ice-cream, dairy (milk fat)	700	170	25	▲					△			○
non-dairy	700	170	21	▲					△			●
Jam, ordinary	1100	260	69			△						
"Jam slimming" (fruit/sugar conserve)	590	140	35									
Jellabi	1300	300	50	△								○
Jelly cubes	1100	260	63			△						
made up with water	250	60	15									
made with milk	360	90	16	△								
Kedgeree	600	140	10	△		△						●
Kidney, lamb, fried	650	150	0	▲		▲	△	▲	▲	▲	▲	●
Kidney, ox, stewed	700	170	0	▲		▲	▲	▲	▲	△	▲	●
Kidney, pig, stewed	650	160	0	▲		▲	△	▲	▲	▲	▲	●
Kipper, baked	900	210	0	▲	△				△		△	●
weighed with bones	450	110	0	△					△		△	●
Ladies fingers, raw	70	17	0		△	△		▲				
canned	65	15	0		△	▲						
Lager, *see* Beer												
Lamb, fat	2500	600	0	△		△			△		△	●
breast, roast	1700	400	0	▲		△			△		△	●
lean only	1000	250	0	▲		△			△	△	▲	●
Lamb, leg, roast	1100	260	0	▲		▲			△	△	▲	●
lean only	800	190	0	▲		▲			▲	△	▲	●

Table 1 (per 100 g) continued

	Kilojoules	Kilocalories	Carbohydrate	Protein	Calcium	Iron	Vitamin A	Vitamin C	Riboflavin	Thiamin	Niacin	Fat
Lamb, loin chop, grilled	1500	360	0	▲		△			△	△	▲	●
weighed with bone	1100	260	0	▲		△			△			●
lean only	900	210	0	▲		△			△	△	▲	●
Lamb, scrag end and neck, stewed	1200	290	0	▲		▲			△		△	●
lean only	1000	240	0	▲		▲			△		△	●
Lamb, shoulder, roast	1300	310	0	▲		△			△		△	●
lean only	800	200	0	▲		△			△	△	△	●
Lamb cutlets, grilled	1500	370	0	▲		△			△	△	▲	●
weighed with bone	1000	240	0	△		△					△	●
lean only	900	220	0	▲	.	△			△	△	▲	●
Lard	3700	900	0									●
Laverbread, cooked, coated with oatmeal	200	50	0			▲		△				
Leek, raw	130	30	0	.	△	△		▲				
boiled	100	25	0		△	△		▲				.
Leek and tomato soup *	100	25	5	△				▲				
Lemon, whole	65	15	0		▲			▲				
Lemonade, bottled or canned	90	20	6									
Lemon curd (made with eggs and lemons)	1200	290	40			△	△					●
shop-bought (starch-based)	1200	290	63									
Lemon juice	50	7	0					▲				
Lemon sole, fried	900	210	10	△	△	△					△	●
weighed with skin and bones	700	170	7	△	△	△					△	●
Lemon sole, steamed	380	90	0	▲							△	
weighed with skin and bones	270	60	0	△							△	
Lentils, raw	1300	300	50	▲		▲			△	▲	△	
cooked	400	100	17	△		▲				△		
Lettuce	50	12	0			▲	▲					
Lime, whole	65	15	0		▲			▲				
Lime juice	30	7	0					▲				
Liquorice allsorts	1300	300	74		△	▲						
Litchis, see Lychées												
Liver, calf, fried	1000	240	0	▲		▲	▲	▲	▲	△	▲	●
Liver, chicken, fried	800	190	0	▲		▲	▲	▲	▲	▲	.	●
Liver, lamb, fried	1000	240	0	▲		▲	▲	▲	▲	△	▲	●
Liver, ox, stewed	800	190	0	▲		▲	▲	▲	▲	△	▲	●
Liver, pig, stewed	800	190	0	▲		▲	▲	▲	▲	△	▲	●
Liver, "tarragon wine" *	570	135	0	▲		▲	▲	▲	▲	△	▲	●
Liver pâté, chicken- *	400	95	0	△		▲	▲	▲	▲	△	△	●
Lobster, boiled	500	120	0	▲	△							○
weighed with shell	180	40	0	△								○
Loganberries, raw	75	18	0			△		▲				
stewed without sugar	70	15	0			△		▲				
with sugar	230	55	13			△		▲				
canned in syrup	440	100	26			△		▲				

Table 1 Lu-Mi

Key △ = 10% RDA
▲ = 25% RDA
○ = 20+ % fat
● = 40+ % fat

	Kilojoules	Kilocalories	Carbohydrate	Protein	Calcium	Iron	Vitamin A	Vitamin C	Riboflavin	Thiamin	Niacin	Fat
Lucozade	290	70	18									
Lychées, raw	270	65	16					▲				
canned	300	70	18					▲				
Macaroni, raw	1600	370	79	△		△				△	△	
boiled	500	120	25									
Macaroni cheese ●	525	125	14	△	▲							●
Mackerel, fried	800	190	0	▲		△			△		▲	●
weighed with bones	600	140	0	▲					△		▲	●
Mackerel pâté ●	670	160	0	▲	△		△	△	△		▲	●
Maize (sweetcorn), boiled	520	120	23			△			△		△	△
Maize grits, raw	1500	360	78	△		△	△			△		
Maize oil	3700	900	0									●
Mandarine oranges, *see* Tangerines												
Mango, raw	250	60	15				▲	▲				
canned	330	80	20				▲	▲				
Margarine	3000	730	0				▲					●
Marmalade	1100	260	70					▲				
Marrow, boiled	30	7	0									
Marrow, stuffed with beef ●	780	190	0	▲	▲	△			△		△	●
Marrow, stuffed with chicken ●	630	150	0	▲	▲			△	△		▲	●
Marzipan	1800	430	50	△	△	△			▲	△		
Matzo	1600	380	87	△		△						
Mayonnaise	3000	700	0									●
Meat, luncheon, canned	1300	310	10	△		△					△	●
Meat paste	700	170	0	△	△	△				△	△	●
Medlars, raw	180	40	10									
Melon, cantaloupe, flesh only (orange-coloured)	100	25	5				▲	▲				
weighed with skin	60	15	0				▲	▲				
Melon, honeydew (yellow)	90	20	5					▲				
weighed with skin	60	15	0					▲				
Melon, watermelon	90	20	5					△				
weighed with skin	60	15	0									
Meringues (without cream)	1600	380	96						△			
Milk, condensed, whole, sweetened	1360	322	56	△	▲		△		▲			○
skimmed, sweetened	1140	270	60	△	▲				▲	△		
Milk, cow's, whole	270	65	4.7		▲				△			●
semi-skim, 2% fat	225	51	4.9		▲				△			○
skimmed	142	33	5		▲				△			
Milk, goat's	300	70	4.6		▲							●
Milk, whole, dried	2050	490	39	▲	▲		▲	▲	▲	▲		●
skimmed, dried	1500	360	53	▲	▲			△	▲	▲		
Millet flour	1480	350	75			△			△	▲	△	
Mincemeat	1200	280	60			△						
Mince pies	1800	430	62		△	△	△				△	●

Table 1 (per 100 g) *continued*

	Kilojoules	Kilocalories	Carbohydrate	Protein	Calcium	Iron	Vitamin A	Vitamin C	Riboflavin	Thiamin	Niacin	Fat
Moules marinières •	420	100	0	△	▲	▲		▲				
Muesli	1550	370	66	△	▲	▲			△	▲	△	
Mulberries, raw	150	35	8			△		▲				
Mushrooms, French •	320	75	0			▲			△		△	●
Mushrooms, raw	50	12	0			△		▲			△	
fried	850	200	0			△		▲			△	●
Mustard and cress	50	10	0	△	△	△	▲					
Nectarines, raw	220	50	12			△	△					
weighed with stones	200	45	11			△	△					
Noodles, wheat, egg, raw	1650	390	72	△		△				△	△	
cooked	510	120	22									
Noodles, wheat, raw	1650	390	76	△		△				▲	△	
cooked	510	120	24							△		
Nuts, *see* named types												
Oatcakes	1850	440	63	△	△	▲				▲		●
Oatmeal, raw	1700	400	73	△	△	▲				▲		○
porridge	190	45	8									
Oil, vegetable	3700	900	0									●
Okra, raw	70	17	0		△	△	▲					
canned	65	15	0		△	▲						
Olive oil	3700	900	0									●
Olives, pickled, flesh only	420	100	0			△						
weighed with stones	340	80	0									
Omelet, basic •	840	200	0	△	△	△	▲		▲			●
Omelet, beef and asparagus •	530	125	0	△		△	△		△			●
Omelet, cheese and tomato •	610	145	0	▲	△	△	△	△	△			●
Omelet, chicken •	760	180	0	▲		△	△		▲		△	●
Omelet, fines herbes •	840	200	0	△	△	△	▲		▲			●
Omelet, lemon soufflé •	590	140	0	△	△	△	△	▲	△			●
Omelet, shrimp •	710	170	0	△	▲	△	△		△			●
Omelet, Spanish •	250	60	0			△	△		△			●
Onions, raw	100	24	5					▲				
boiled	50	12	3					△				
fried	1400	340	10	△								●
spring, raw	150	35	9	▲	△			▲				
Orange, flesh only	170	40	10			△	▲					
weighed with peel	130	30	8			△	▲					
juice	170	40	10			△	▲					
Orange juice, canned, unsweetened	170	40	10			△	▲					
sweetened	190	45	12			△	▲					
made from concentrate, unsweetened	170	40	10			△	▲					
Oxtail, stewed	400	95	0	△		△			△		△	●
meat only	1000	240	0	▲		▲			△		△	●
Pancake, Scotch •	1000	250	17	△	▲	△			△	△		

Table 1

Key △ = 10% RDA
▲ = 25% RDA
○ = 20+ % fat
● = 40+ % fat

	Kilojoules	Kilocalories	Carbohydrate	Protein	Calcium	Iron	Vitamin A	Vitamin C	Riboflavin	Thiamin	Niacin	Fat
Pancakes	1300	310	36		▲	△				△	△	●
Papadum, raw	1200	290	46	▲	△	▲					△	
Papaya, *see* Paw paw												
Parsley, raw	90	20	0		▲	▲	▲	▲	△	△		
Parsnip, boiled	240	60	14				▲					
Partridge, roast, with bone	500	120	0	▲		▲			▲	▲	▲	○
without bone	900	220	0	▲		▲			▲	▲	▲	○
Passion fruit, pulp only	150	35	6			△		▲				
weighed whole	60	15	3					▲				
Pastilles	1100	260	62			△						
Pastry, choux, raw	900	220	20		△	△	△			△	△	●
cooked	1400	330	30	△	△	△	▲			△	△	●
Pastry, flaky, raw	1800	430	36		△	△	△				△	●
cooked	2400	570	47		△	△	▲				△	●
Pastry, shortcrust, raw	1900	460	48		△	△	△				△	●
cooked	2200	520	56		△	△	△				△	●
Pâté, mackerel ●	670	160	0	△	△			△	△		▲	●
Paw paw, fresh	170	40	10			△		▲				
canned	280	70	15			△		▲				
Peach	160	40	9				▲	△				
weighed with stone	140	35	8				▲	△				
Peach, canned without sugar	190	45	10				△					
in syrup	370	90	23				△					
Peach, dried, uncooked	900	210	50			▲	▲		△		▲	
stewed without sugar	340	80	20			▲	▲				△	
with sugar	400	95	23			▲	▲				△	
Peanut butter	2600	620	13	▲	△	△				▲	▲	●
Peanuts, fresh	2400	570	9	▲	△	△				▲	▲	●
roasted	2400	570	9	▲	△	△				▲	▲	●
Pear, canned in water	130	30	8									
in syrup	330	80	20									
Pear, cooking	130	30	8									
stewed without sugar	130	30	8									
with sugar	280	65	17									
Peas, dried, boiled	440	100	18	△		△				△		
Peas, garden, canned	200	50	7			△		△		△	△	
processed	340	80	14			△						
Peas, raw	280	70	11			△	△	▲		▲	△	
boiled	220	50	8			△	△	▲		△	△	
frozen	220	50	7			△	△	▲		▲	△	
boiled	180	40	4			△	△	△		△	△	
Peas, split, boiled	500	120	22	△		△				△		
Pepper, green, raw	65	15	0				△	▲				
boiled	60	14	0				△	▲				
Peppermints	1700	400	100									

99

Table 1 (per 100 g) continued Ph-Po	Kilojoules	Kilocalories	Carbohydrate	Protein	Calcium	Iron	Vitamin A	Vitamin C	Riboflavin	Thiamin	Niacin	Fat
Pheasant, whole, roasted	550	130	0	▲		▲					△	●
without bone	900	220	0	▲		▲				△	▲	●
Pickle, piccalilli	140	30	0									
sweet	570	130	0		△							
Pie, fruit, individual	1600	380	57	△	△							●
pastry top	750	180	28	△				△				●
Pie, lemon meringue	1400	330	46	△	△	△	△					●
Pigeon, roast	420	100	0	△		▲					△	●
meat only	1000	240	0	▲		▲					▲	●
Pilchards, canned in tomato sauce	500	120	0	▲	▲	▲			△		▲	●
Pineapple, fresh	190	45	12					▲				
canned in water	190	45	12					▲				
in syrup	330	80	20					▲				
Pitta, white (bread)	1100	260	58	△	△	△				△		
Plaice, fried in batter	1200	290	15	△	△	△			△	△	△	●
crumbs	1000	240	10	▲	△				△	△	△	●
Plaice, steamed	400	100	0	▲					△	△	△	
weighed with bones	200	50	0	△								
Plantain, green, raw	500	120	30					▲				
boiled	500	120	30									
ripe, fried	1100	270	50					△				○
Plums, cooking, raw	110	30	6					△				
weighed with stones	100	25	6					△				
Plums, stewed without sugar	90	22	5					△				
weighed with stones	85	20	5					△				
Plums, dessert	160	40	10					△				
weighed with stones	150	35	9					△				
Plums, stewed with sugar	250	60	15									
weighed with stones	230	55	14									
Plums, stewed without sugar	90	20	5									
weighed with stones	85	19	5									
Polony	1200	290	15	△		△				△		●
Pomegranate juice	190	45	12					△				
Popcorn, unpopped	1510	360	72	△		△				△	△	
popped, plain	1600	380	77	△		△				△	△	
sugar-coated	1600	380	85									
Pork, leg, roast	1200	290	0	▲		△			△	▲	▲	●
lean only	800	180	0	▲		△			▲	▲	▲	●
Pork chops, grilled	1400	330	0	▲		△			▲	▲	▲	●
weighed with bone	1100	260	0	▲		△			△	▲	▲	●
lean only, weighed with fat and bone	550	130	0	▲					△	▲	▲	○
Pork pie (50% meat)	1500	360	25	△	△	△				△	△	●
Potato, dried powder	1400	330	73	△	△	▲		▲			▲	
made up	300	70	16									

Table 1   Po-Ri

Key △ = 10% RDA
 ▲ = 25% RDA
 ○ = 20+ % fat
 ● = 40+ % fat

	Kilojoules	Kilocalories	Carbohydrate	Protein	Calcium	Iron	Vitamin A	Vitamin C	Riboflavin	Thiamin	Niacin	Fat
Potato, new, boiled	320	75	18					▲				
canned	220	50	13					▲				
Potato, old, boiled	340	80	20					△				
mashed (with margarine and milk)	500	120	18					△				○
baked, with skin	360	85	20					△				
Potato, roast	660	160	27					△				○
chips	1000	240	40					△				○
frozen chips	460	110	20					△				
fried	1200	290	29					△				
Potato, sweet, boiled	360	85	20				▲	▲				
Potato crisps	2200	530	50			△		▲		△	△	●
Prawns, boiled	450	110	0	▲	▲	△						
weighed with shell	170	40	0	△	△							
Prunes, dried, uncooked	700	170	40			▲		△				
weighed with stones	600	140	35			▲		△				
Prunes, stewed with sugar	450	110	25			△						
weighed with stones	400	100	24			△						
Prunes, stewed without sugar	350	80	20			△						
weighed with stones	320	75	19			△						
Pudding, black, fried	1300	300	15	△		▲						●
Pudding, sponge, steamed	1450	350	46	▲	△	△						●
Pudding, suet, steamed	1400	330	40	▲	△							●
Puffa Puffa Rice (Kellogg's)	1720	410	83			▲			▲	▲	▲	
Puffed Wheat (Quaker)	1400	330	69	△		▲					▲	
Pumpkin, raw	65	15	0				▲	△				
cooked	80	20	0				▲	△				
Quince, raw	100	25	6					▲				
Rabbit, stewed, with bones	400	100	0	△		△					△	●
meat	750	180	0	▲					△		△	●
Radishes	65	15	0		△	△		▲				
Raisins	1000	250	65		△	△						
Raspberries, raw	100	25	6			△		▲				
stewed without sugar	100	25	6			△		▲				
with sugar	300	70	17			△		▲				
canned	370	90	23			△		△				
Ready Brek (Lyons)	1650	390	70	△	△	▲				▲	▲	
Rhubarb, raw	25	6	0		△			△				
stewed without sugar	25	6	0		△			△				
with sugar	200	50	12		△			△				
canned in syrup	200	50	12		△			△				
Ribena	1000	230	60					▲				
Rice, boil-in-bag (Kellogg's)	1370	330	76	△								
boiled	520	125	30									
Rice, brown, raw	1520	355	81			△				▲	▲	

Table 1 (per 100 g) continued

	Kilojoules	Kilocalories	Carbohydrate	Protein	Calcium	Iron	Vitamin A	Vitamin C	Riboflavin	Thiamin	Niacin	Fat
boiled	520	125	30									
Rice, parboiled, raw	1520	360	79	△		△				△	△	
cooked	520	125	30									
Rice, white, raw	1540	360	87	△							△	
Rice flour	1530	370	80		△						△	
Rice Krispies (Kellogg's)	1440	350	84		▲				▲	▲	▲	
Rice pudding, canned	400	95	15		△				△			○
Ricicles (Kellogg's)	1470	350	88		▲				▲	▲	▲	
Roe, cod, hard, fried	850	200	0	▲		△	△		▲	▲		●
herring, soft, fried	1000	240	0	▲		△			▲	△	△	●
Rose-hip syrup	1000	230	60					▲				
Rye flour	1430	340	76	△		▲			△	▲		
Safflower-seed oil	3700	900	0									●
Sago, raw	1520	360	94		△							
boiled	500	120	31									
Salad cream	1300	300	15									●
Salami	2000	480	0	▲		△			△	△	▲	●
Salmon, canned	650	155	0	▲	△	△	△		△		▲	
smoked	600	140	0	▲					△	△	▲	○
Salmon, steamed	800	190	0	▲						△	▲	●
weighed with bones	650	150	0	△						△	▲	●
Salsify, boiled	80	20	0		△	△		△				
Samosas (minced lamb)	2400	570	9			△					△	●
Sardines, canned with oil, drained	900	220	0	▲	▲	▲			▲		▲	●
canned in tomato sauce	750	180	0	△	▲	▲				△	▲	●
Sauce, brown	420	100	25		▲	△						
tomato	360	90	8				▲	△				●
ketchup	420	100	24		△		▲					
Sausage, beef, fried	1100	260	15	△	△	△					▲	●
Sausage, beef, grilled	1100	260	15	△	△	△					▲	●
Sausage, liver	1300	300	5	△		▲	▲		▲	△	△	●
Sausage, pork, grilled	1300	300	10	△	△	△				△	△	●
Sausage, pork, fried	1300	300	10	△	△	△				△	△	●
Sausage roll, flaky pastry	2000	480	35	△	△	△				△	△	●
Sausage roll, short pastry	1900	450	35	△	△	△				△	△	●
Saveloy	1000	240	10	△		△					△	○
Scallops, steamed, without shells	450	100	0	▲	▲	▲						
Scampi, fried in breadcrumbs	130	30	30									●
Scones	1560	370	56	△	▲	△	△					○
Scones, drop *	1100	270	12	△	▲	▲	▲		△	△	△	○
Scotch pancakes	1200	285	40	△	▲	△	△					○
Seakale, boiled	30	8	0		△			▲				
Semolina, raw	1490	350	78	△		△					△	
boiled	500	120	31									
pudding, canned	390	90	15									

Table 1   Sh-Su

Key △ = 10% RDA ▲ = 25% RDA ○ = 20+ % fat ● = 40+ % fat	Kilojoules	Kilocalories	Carbohydrate	Protein	Calcium	Iron	Vitamin A	Vitamin C	Riboflavin	Thiamin	Niacin	Fat
Sherry, dry	480	115	0									
medium	490	116	4									
sweet	570	135	7									
Shortbread	2000	475	66	△	△	△	▲			△		●
Shredded Wheat (Nabisco)	1400	330	68	△		▲				▲	▲	
Shrimp omelet ●	710	170	0	△	▲	△	△		△			●
Shrimp surprise ●	150	35	0	△	△			▲				
Shrimps, boiled	500	120	0	▲	▲	△					△	
weighed with shell	160	40	0	△	△							
canned	400	90	0	▲	△	▲						
Shrimps in tomatoes ●	420	100	10	△	▲	△		▲		△		○
Skate, fried in batter	850	200	5	▲	△	△					△	●
fried in batter with skin and bones	700	170	4	△							△	●
Smacks (Kellogg's)	1530	370	87	△		△			▲	▲	▲	
Soup, celery ●	90	22	3		△							
Soup, leek and tomato ●	100	25	5		△			▲				
Soup, watercress and yogurt ●	180	43	5		▲			△	△			
Soyabean oil	3700	900	0									●
Soyabeans, raw	1700	400	30	▲	▲	▲			△	▲	△	●
Soya curd, steamed	290	70	0	△	▲	△						●
Soya flour, full-fat	1870	450	24	▲	▲	▲			△	▲	△	●
low-fat	1490	350	28	▲	▲	▲			▲	▲	△	
Spaghetti, raw	1600	375	84	△		△				△	△	
boiled	500	120	26									
canned in tomato sauce	250	60	12									
Special K (Kellogg's)	1500	360	73	▲	△	▲			▲	▲	▲	
Spinach, boiled	130	30	0		▲	▲	▲	▲				
Sprats, fried	1800	430	0	▲	▲	▲			△		▲	●
weighed with bones	1600	380	0	▲	▲	▲					△	●
Spreads, low-fat	1500	370	0				▲					●
Spring greens, boiled	40	10	0		△	△	▲	▲	△			
Squash, raw	100	25	5			△	△	▲				
Steak, stewed with gravy, canned	750	180	1	△		△					△	●
Steak-and-kidney pie	1200	290	15	△		▲	△		▲	▲	△	●
Stout, *see* Beer												
Strawberries	100	25	6					▲				
canned in syrup	350	80	20					▲				
Suet	3700	900	0									●
Sugar, brown	1680	395	100									
cubes	1680	395	100									
icing	1680	395	100									
white granulated	1680	395	100									
Sugar confectionery, *see* specific types												
Sugar Puffs (Quaker)	1500	350	85			△			△			

103

Table 1
(per 100 g)
continued   Su-Ve

	Kilojoules	Kilocalories	Carbohydrate	Protein	Calcium	Iron	Vitamin A	Vitamin C	Riboflavin	Thiamin	Niacin	Fat
Sultana Bran (Kellogg's)	1300	310	69	△	△	▲			▲	▲	▲	
Sultanas	1000	250	65		△	△						
Swedes, boiled	80	20	0		△			▲				
Sweetbread, lamb, fried	1000	240	10	▲		△		▲	△		△	●
Sweetcorn, boiled	520	120	23				△	△		△	△	
Sweetcorn, canned	320	80	16				△	△				
Sweet potatoes, boiled	360	80	16				▲	▲				
Sweets, *see* specific types												
Sweets, boiled	1400	330	87									
Syrup, golden	1270	300	79									
Tangerine, flesh only	170	40	10				△	▲				
weighed with peel	130	30	8				△	▲				
juice	170	40	10				△	▲				
Tangerine juice, canned, unsweetened	170	40	10				△	▲				
sweetened	190	45	12				△	▲				
Tapioca, raw	1530	360	95									
Taramasalata	1800	430	4									●
Tarts, jam	1600	380	63		△	△						○
Toffees	1800	430	70									
Tofu, canned, fried	1300	300	4	▲	▲	▲						●
Tofu, steamed	290	70	0	△	▲	△						●
Tomato, canned	50	12	0				△	▲				
Tomato, raw	60	14	0				▲	▲				
fried	300	70	0									●
Tomato juice, canned	70	17	0				△	▲				
Tomato sauce	360	90	8				▲	△				●
ketchup	420	100	24		△		▲					
Tongue, canned	900	210	0	△		▲			▲		△	●
Tongue, ox, pickled	1200	290	0	▲		▲			△		△	●
Tongue, sheep, stewed	1200	290	0	▲		▲		△	▲	△	△	●
Treacle	1100	260	67		▲	▲						
Treacle tart	1600	380	61		△	△						○
Trifle	700	170	25		△							○
Tripe, stewed	400	100	0	△	▲							●
Trout, steamed	600	140	0	▲		△			△		△	○
weighed with bones	400	100	0	▲					△		△	○
Tuna, canned in oil, drained	1200	290	0	▲		△			△		▲	●
Turkey, roast	700	170	0	▲		△			△		▲	
meat only	600	140	0	▲		△			△		▲	
light meat	550	130	0	▲					△		▲	
dark meat	600	140	0	▲		△			△		▲	○
Turnip, boiled	60	14	0		△		△	▲				
Turnip tops, boiled	50	12	0		△	▲	▲	▲				
Veal, jellied, canned	500	120	0	▲		△			△		▲	○

Table 1

Key △ = 10% RDA
△ ▲ = 25% RDA
○ = 20+ % fat
● = 40+ % fat

	Kilojoules	Kilocalories	Carbohydrate	Protein	Calcium	Iron	Vitamin A	Vitamin C	Riboflavin	Thiamin	Niacin	Fat
Veal and mushrooms *	380	90	4	△	△				△		▲	○
Veal cutlet, fried in egg and breadcrumbs	900	200	0	▲		△			△		▲	○
fillet, roast	950	220	0	▲		△			△		▲	●
Veal pimentos *	190	45	4			△	△	▲	△		△	○
Venison, roast	800	200	0	▲		▲			△		△	○
Vermouth, dry	500	120	6									
sweet	630	150	16									
Vodka	920	220	0									
Walnuts	2200	530	5	△	△	△				△		●
Watercress	60	14	0		▲	△	▲	▲				
Watercress and yogurt soup *	180	43	5		▲				△	△		
Watermelon, *see* Melon, water												
Weetabix	1450	340	70	△		▲			▲	▲	▲	
Wheatgerm oil	3700	900	0									●
Whelks, boiled (without shells)	400	100	0	▲	△	▲						
Whisky	920	220	0									
Whitebait, fried	2000	480	0	▲	▲	▲			△		▲	●
Whiting, fried	800	190	7	▲	△				△	△	△	●
weighed with bones	700	180	6	▲	△				△	△	△	●
Wine, port	660	160	12									
Wine, red	280	70	0									
white, dry	280	70	0									
medium	310	75	0									
sweet	400	95	0									
Winkles, boiled (without shells)	300	70	0	△	▲	▲						
Yam, boiled	500	120	0									
Yogurt, low-fat, unflavoured	220	50	6		▲				△			
flavoured	400	90	16		▲				△			
Yorkshire pudding	900	210	26	△	▲	△			△	△		●
Zucchini, raw	100	25	5			△	△	▲				

Table 2
Nutritional values per portion

	Kilojoules	Kilocalories	Carbohydrate	Protein	Calcium	Iron	Vitamin A	Vitamin C	Riboflavin	Thiamin	Niacin	Fat
Ackee, canned, 150 g	900	210	0				▲					●
Advocaat liqueur, 50 ml	550	130	14									
Ale, see Beer												
All-Bran (Kellogg's), 30 g + 100 ml full-cream milk	580	140	19		△	△			△	△	△	○
+ semi-skimmed milk (2% fat)	540	130	23		△	△			△	△	△	
Almonds, 30 g	750	180	0		△				△			●
Anchovies, canned, drained, 50 g	600	150	0	△	△	△						●
Apple, one	200	50	15									
Apple, baked with sugar, one	340	80	20									
stewed with sugar, 150 g	340	80	20									
without sugar, 150 g	200	50	15									
Apple crumble (180 g)	1600	375	67									○
Apple snow *	380	90	14									
Apricots, canned in syrup, 150 g	700	170	45				▲					
Apricots, dried, stewed with sugar, 150 g	530	130	30				▲					
without sugar, 150 g	450	100	23				▲					
Apricots, raw, with stones, 150 g	150	35	9				▲	△				
Apricots, stewed with sugar, with stones, 150 g	360	80	23				▲	△				
stewed with sugar, without stones, 150 g	150	35	16				▲	△				
stewed without sugar, without stones, 150 g	150	35	9				▲	△				
Artichoke, globe, boiled, 150 g	45	10	0									
Artichoke, Jerusalem, boiled, 150 g	120	30	0									
Aubergine, raw, 150 g	90	20	0									
Aubergine stuffed with beef *	1700	400	3.5	▲	▲	△		△	△		△	●
Aubergine stuffed with chicken*	1260	300	3	▲	▲			△	△		▲	●
Avocado pears, 150 g	1350	320	0			△		▲				●
Bacon, back, fried, 100 g	1900	460	0	△						△	△	●
middle	2000	480	0	△						△	△	●
streaky	2000	480	0	△						△	△	●
Bacon, back, grilled, 100 g	1700	400	0	△						△	△	●
middle	1700	400	0	△						△	△	●
streaky	1750	420	0	△						△	△	●
Bacon, collar joint, 100 g	1350	330	0	△						△	△	●
lean only	800	200	0	△						△	△	●
Bacon, gammon joint, 100 g	1110	270	0	△						△	△	●
lean only, 100 g	700	170	0	△						△	△	●
Bamboo shoots, canned, 100 g	100	25	4									
Banana, 150 g	530	130	30					▲				
Barcelona nuts, 30 g	900	220	0									●
Barley, cooked, 150 g	750	180	42									
Barley, whole grain, 100 g	1400	330	69			▲				△	△	

Table 2 Be-Be

Key △ = ⅙ RDA
▲ = ½ RDA
○ = 20+ % fat
● = 40+ % fat

	Kilojoules	Kilocalories	Carbohydrate	Protein	Calcium	Iron	Vitamin A	Vitamin C	Riboflavin	Thiamin	Niacin	Fat
boiled, 100 g	470	110	23		△						△	
Beans, broad, boiled, 150 g	300	70	10		△			▲			△	
butter, boiled, 150 g	600	150	25		△					▲	△	
French, boiled, 150 g	45	10	0				△	△				
haricot, boiled, 150 g	600	150	25	△	△					▲	△	
haricot, canned in tomato sauce, 200 g	540	120	20	△	△							
mung, cooked, 150 g	700	150	17		△							
runner, boiled, 150 g	120	30	0				△	△				
valor, canned, 150 g	120	30	0									
Beansprouts, canned, 150 g	60	15	0									
Beef, corned, canned, 200 g	1800	420	0	▲		▲			△		△	●
Beef, curried, 200 g	1400	330	15	△		▲						●
Beef, rump steak, fried, 200 g	2000	480	0	▲		▲			△		▲	●
lean only	1600	380	0	▲		▲			▲		▲	●
Beef, rump steak, grilled, 200 g	1800	440	0	▲		▲			△		▲	●
lean only	1400	340	0	▲		▲			▲		▲	●
Beef, silverside, boiled, 200 g	2000	480	0	▲		▲			△		△	●
lean only	1500	360	0	▲		▲			△		△	○
Beef, sirloin, roast, 200 g	2400	580	0	▲		▲			△		△	●
lean only	1600	380	0	▲		▲			△		△	●
Beef, spiced •	1470	350	4	△		△		▲			△	●
Beef, stewing steak, 200 g	1800	420	0	▲		▲			△		△	●
Beef, topside, roast, 200 g	1800	420	0	▲		▲			△		▲	●
lean only	1300	300	0	▲		▲			△		▲	●
Beef brisket, 200 g	2700	660	0	▲		▲			△		▲	●
Beef forerib, roast, 200 g	3000	760	0	▲		△			△		△	●
lean only	1800	440	0	▲		▲			△		▲	●
Beef goulash •	1260	300	22	△	▲	△		△	△	△	△	○
Beef mince, stewed, 200 g	2000	480	0	▲		▲			△		▲	●
Beef steak pudding, 200 g	2000	480	40	△	△	△					△	●
Beef stew, 200 g	1000	240	10	△		△	▲				△	●
Beef-stuffed aubergine •	1700	400	3.5	▲	▲	△			△		△	●
Beef and vegetable stew •	920	220	5	△		△	△	△	△		△	●
Beer, ale, pale, bottled, 500 ml	675	160	10									
Beer, bitter, draught, 500 ml	650	150	11									
Beer, bitter, keg, 500 ml	650	150	11									
Beer, brown ale, 500 ml	600	150	15									
Beer, canned, bitter, 500 ml	650	150	10									
Beer, lager, bottled, 500 ml	600	150	8									
Beer, mild, draught, 500 ml	500	125	10									
Beer, stout, bottled, 500 ml	780	185	10									
extra, 500 ml	820	195	10									
strong ale, 500 ml	1500	360	30									
Beetroot, boiled, 150 g	300	70	15					△				

Table 2
(per portion)
continued
Be-Ca

	Kilojoules	Kilocalories	Carbohydrate	Protein	Calcium	Iron	Vitamin A	Vitamin C	Riboflavin	Thiamin	Niacin	Fat
Bengal gram, cooked, 200 g	1200	290	44	△	△	▲	△			△		
Bilberries, raw, 150 g	380	90	23					▲				
Blackberries, raw, 150 g	190	45	10		△			▲				
stewed without sugar, 150 g	170	40	10		△			▲				
with sugar, 150 g	380	90	25		△			▲				
Bloater, grilled, 200 g	2000	480	0	▲	▲	▲			△		△	●
weighed with bones	1600	380	0	▲	△	△					△	●
Brain, calf, boiled, 200 g	1300	300	0	△		△			△		△	●
Brain, lamb, 200 g	1000	240	0	△		△			△	△	△	●
Brandy, 50 ml	460	110	0									
Brandy and soda, 150 ml	460	110	0									
Bran Buds (Kellogg's), 30 g + 100 ml full-cream milk	590	140	20		△	△			△	△	△	○
+ semi-skimmed milk	545	130	20		△	△			△	△	△	
Bran Flakes (Kellogg's), 30 g + 100 ml full cream milk	670	160	25		△	△			△	△	△	○
+ semi-skimmed milk	620	150	25		△	△			△	△	△	
Brawn, 200 g	1200	290	0	△		△						
Brazil nuts, 30 g	750	180	0							△		●
Bread, brown, 2 slices = 60 g	570	130	27									
toasted, 2 slices = 50 g	630	150	32									
white, 2 slices = 60 g	600	140	30									
wholemeal, 2 slices = 60 g	550	130	25									
Bread, West Indian, 2 slices	720	300	35	△								
Bread-and-butter pudding, 180 g	1200	290	30	▲			△		△			●
Broccoli tops, boiled, 150 g	120	30	0		△		▲	▲	△			
Brussels sprouts, raw, 150 g	150	40	0				△	▲				
boiled, 150 g	100	25	0				△	▲				
Butter, 15 g	460	110	0				△					●
Cabbage, red, raw, 150 g	130	30	0		△			▲				
Savoy, raw, 150 g	150	35	0		△		△	▲				
spring, boiled, 150 g	45	10	0				△	▲				
white, raw, 150 g	120	30	0					▲				
winter, raw, 150 g	120	30	0		△			▲				
winter, boiled, 150 g	100	25	0					▲				
Cakes, Chinese rice flour, 100 g	1200	300	60									
Carrots, canned, 150 g	120	30	6				▲	△				
old, raw, 150 g	150	40	7		△		▲	△				
boiled, 150 g	120	30	6				▲	△				
young, boiled, 150 g	140	35	6				▲	△				
Cauliflower, raw, 150 g	90	20	0					▲				
boiled, 150 g	60	15	0					▲				
Cauliflower cheese, 150 g	700	170	7	▲								●
Cauliflower cheese *	670	160	8	△				▲	△			●

Table 2

Key △ = $\frac{1}{6}$ RDA
   ▲ = $\frac{1}{2}$ RDA
   ○ = 20+ % fat
   ● = 40+ % fat

	Kilojoules	Kilocalories	Carbohydrate	Protein	Calcium	Iron	Vitamin A	Vitamin C	Riboflavin	Thiamin	Niacin	Fat
Celeriac, boiled, 150 g	60	15	0		△							
Celery, raw, 150 g	60	15	0		△			△				
boiled, 150 g	30	7	0		△			△				
Celery soup *	420	100	14	▲				△	△			
Cheese, cauliflower *	670	160	8	△				▲	△			●
Cheese, macaroni *	1550	370	42	△	▲			△	△			●
Cheesecake, 180 g	3200	770	45		△		▲					●
Cheese soufflé, 150 g	1500	380	15	△	▲		△		△			●
Cherries, glacé, 20 g	180	40	11									
Cherries, raw, with stones, 150 g	260	60	15					△				
without stones, 150 g	300	75	18					△				
Cherries, stewed with sugar, weighed with stones, 150 g	450	100	27									
without stones, 150 g	500	120	30									
Cherries, stewed without sugar, weighed with stones, 150 g	210	50	12									
without stones, 150 g	260	60	15									
Cherry brandy, 50 ml	550	130	16									
Chestnuts, 30 g	200	50	10									
Chevda, 50 g	825	200	14			△				△	△	○
Chicken, curried, mayonnaise *	1260	300	4	▲		△		▲	△	△	▲	○
Chicken curry *	840	200	6	△	△	△		△	△	△	△	○
Chicken, roast with skin, 200 g	1800	430	0	▲							▲	●
meat only	1250	300	0	▲					△		▲	○
light meat	1200	280	0	▲							▲	○
dark meat	1300	300	0	▲		△			△		▲	○
Chicken, spiced, grilled *	1100	260	0	△							△	●
Chicken-stuffed aubergine *	1260	300	3	▲	▲			△	△		▲	●
Chicken leg, weighed with bone	400	100	0	△							△	○
wing, weighed with bone	150	40	0									○
Chicken-liver pâté *	550	130	0	△		▲	▲	▲	▲		△	●
Chicken omelet *	1200	290	0	△		△	△		△		△	●
Chicken salad *	840	200	3	▲	△			△	△	△	▲	○
Chickpeas, cooked, 200 g	1200	290	44	△	△	▲				△		
Chicory, raw, 150 g	60	15	0				△					
Chocolate, *Bounty* bar, 100 g	2000	470	58	△								●
Chocolate, drinking, *see* Cocoa												
Chocolate, *Mars* bar, 10 g	1850	440	67	△								●
Chocolate, milk, 100 g	2200	530	60	△								●
plain, 100 g	2200	530	65		△							●
Chocolates, filled, 100 g	1900	450	75	△								●
Chutney, apple, 50 g	400	95	25									
tomato, 50 g	330	80	40									
Cider, dry, 500 ml	760	180	13									
sweet, 500 ml	880	210	22									
vintage 500 ml	2100	510	37									

Table 2
(per portion)
continued

	Kilojoules	Kilocalories	Carbohydrate	Protein	Calcium	Iron	Vitamin A	Vitamin C	Riboflavin	Thiamin	Niacin	Fat
Clementines, *see* Tangerines												
Cobnuts, 30 g	500	120	0									●
Coca-Cola, 200 ml	340	86	21									
Cockles, boiled without shells, 300 g	600	150	0	▲	▲	▲						
Cocoa, made with water + milk and sugar, 200 ml	380	90	12									
all milk, 200 ml	920	220	22		▲		△		△			
drinking chocolate, all milk, 200 ml	1100	260	30		▲		△		△			
Coconut, 30 g	500	120	0									●
desiccated, 30 g	750	180	0									●
coconut milk, 200 ml	180	40	10									
Cod, dried, salted, boiled, 200 g	1200	280	0	▲		△						
Cod, smoked, raw, 200 g	700	160	0	▲								
poached, 200 g	860	200	0	▲								
Cod almondesa *	1350	320	0	△	△	△	△	▲	△	△	△	●
Cod fillet, baked, 200 g	800	200	0	▲								
weighed with skin and bones	700	160	0	▲								
Cod fillet, fried, 200 g	1500	360	0	▲								●
fried in batter	1700	400	20	▲								●
Cod fillet, grilled, 200 g	800	200	0	▲								
poached, 200 g	800	200	0	▲								
weighed with bones and skin	700	160	0	▲								
Cod in parsley sauce *	1550	370	42	▲	▲		△	▲	△	△		
Cod liver oil, teaspoon = 5 g	180	45	0				▲					●
Coleslaw salad *	210	50	4				▲	▲				
Compote, apple and orange *	590	140	42					▲				
Compote, plum *	340	80	23									
Consommé with vegetables *	85	20	6				▲	▲				
Cornflakes (Kellogg's), 30 g + 100 ml full-cream milk	700	170	29		△	△			△	△	△	○
+ semi-skimmed milk (2% fat)	660	150	29		△	△			△	△		
Cornish pastie, 300 g	4200	1000	120	△	△	△				△	△	●
Cornmeal, sifted, uncooked, 100 g	1550	370	73			△				△		
unsifted, 100 g	1500	350	72			△				△		
Corn-on-the-cob, 200 g	1000	240	46				△	△		△	△	
Country Store (Kellogg's), 75 g + 100 ml full-cream milk	1380	330	56	△	▲	▲			△	△	▲	○
+ semi-skimmed milk (2% fat)	1330	320	56	△	▲	▲			△	△	▲	
Courgettes, raw, 200 g	200	50	10			▲	△	▲				
Couscous (millet), 100 g	950	230	51			▲				△		
Crab, boiled, 200 g	1100	260	0	▲		△			△	△	△	○
weighed with shell (85% waste), 1000 g	900	200	0	▲		△			△	△	△	○
Crab, canned, 200 g	680	160	0	▲	▲	▲						
Cranberries, raw, 150 g	90	20	0			△		▲				
cooked, sweetened, 150 g	1100	270	70									

Table 2

Key △ = $\frac{1}{6}$ RDA
▲ = $\frac{1}{2}$ RDA
○ = 20+ % fat
● = 40+ % fat

	Kilojoules	Kilocalories	Carbohydrate	Protein	Calcium	Iron	Vitamin A	Vitamin C	Riboflavin	Thiamin	Niacin	Fat
Cranberry sauce, sweetened, 50 g	400	90	25									
Crisps, potato, 50 g	1000	240	25			△		△			△	●
Cucumber, raw, 150 g	60	15	0					△				
Curaçao, 50 ml	650	160	14									
Custard, 100 g	580	140	27	△								○
Custard, egg *	530	125	5	△					△			●
Custard, egg, baked, 150 g	750	180	17	△					△			●
Custard, low-calorie *	340	80	12	△					△			
Custard (from powder), 100 g	500	120	17	△					△			○
Dahl, cooked, 200 g	1200	290	44	△	△	▲	△			△		
Dahl, cooked (from Mung beans), 200 g	900	210	22	△		▲	△					○
Dahl, Masur, cooked (from lentils), 200 g	800	190	22			△						○
Damsons, raw, with stones, 150 g	230	50	15									
without stones, 150 g	240	60	15									
Damsons, stewed with sugar, weighed with stones, 150 g	400	100	26									
without stones, 150 g	440	105	27									
Damsons, stewed without sugar, weighed with stones, 150 g	200	45	10									
without stones, 150 g	210	50	12									
Dates, dried, with stones, 150 g	1350	320	80		△	△					△	
without stones, 150 g	1500	360	100		△	△					△	
Dogfish, fried in batter, 200 g	2200	520	16	△		▲					▲	●
weighed with skin and bones, 200 g	2000	480	14	△		▲					▲	●
Duck, roast, 200 g	2800	680	0	▲		▲			▲	▲	▲	●
meat only, 200 g	1600	380	0	▲		▲			▲	▲	▲	
Dumpling, 50 g	450	110	13	△								●
Eel, stewed, 200 g	1400	360	0	△			▲		△	△	△	●
Egg, duck, one	400	100	0		△	△			△			●
Egg custard *	530	125	5	△					△			●
Eggs, boiled (2)	610	150	0	△			△		△			●
fried (2)	960	230	0	△			△		△			●
omelet (2)	790	190	0	△			△		△			●
poached (2)	640	150	0	△			△		△			●
scrambled (2)	1000	260	0	△			△		△			●
Eggs, scrambled, with asparagus *	970	230	0	△			△	△	△			●
Eggs, scrambled, with smoked salmon *	1100	260	0	△			△		△	△	△	●
Endive, raw, 150 g	75	18	0			▲	▲	▲				
Endive salad *	340	80	0			△	△	△			△	●
Endive and walnut salad *	550	130	0					△				●
Extra (Kellogg's), 30 g + 100 ml full-cream milk	680	160	23	△	△				△	△	△	○
+ semi-skimmed milk (2% fat)	640	150	23	△	△				△	△	△	
Faggots, 200 g	2000	480	30	△	△	▲	▲		▲	△	△	●

**Table 2
(per portion)**
continued

	Kilojoules	Kilocalories	Carbohydrate	Protein	Calcium	Iron	Vitamin A	Vitamin C	Riboflavin	Thiamin	Niacin	Fat
Figs, dried, 150 g	1350	320	75		▲	▲						
stewed without sugar, 150 g	750	180	45		▲	▲						
fresh, 150 g	260	60	15									
Fish cakes, frozen, 100 g	500	120	17	△	△							
fried, 100 g	800	200	17	△								●
Fish fingers, frozen, 100 g	750	180	16	△								○
fried, 100 g	1000	240	17	△								●
Fish paste, 50 g	350	80	2		△	▲						●
Fish pie (with potatoes and milk), 200 g	1000	240	25	△								○
Frankfurters, 200 g	2200	520	6	△		△						●
French dressing, 30 ml	800	200	0									●
Frosties (Kellogg's), 30 g + 100 ml full-cream milk	710	170	31		△	△			△	△	△	○
+ semi-skimmed milk (2% fat)	670	155	36		△	△			△	△	△	
Fruit salad, canned in syrup, 150 g	600	140	40									
Gari, raw (fermented cassava), 100 g	1450	350	83									
Ghee, butter, 15 g	540	130	0									●
vegetable, 15 g	540	130	0									●
Gin, 50 ml	460	110	0									
Gin and soda, 150 ml	460	110	0									
Golden syrup, 15 g	190	45	12									
Gooseberries, dessert, 150 g	230	50	15					▲				
Gooseberries, green, raw, 150 g	100	25	0					▲				
stewed without sugar, 150 g	90	20	0					▲				
with sugar, 150 g	300	75	18					▲				
Gooseberry fool •	670	160	16		▲			▲	△			
Goulash, beef •	1260	300	22	△	▲	△		△	△	△	△	○
Granadilla, pulp only, 100 g	150	35	6					△				
whole fruit, 100 g	60	15	3					△				
Grapefruit, canned in syrup, 150 g	380	90	24					▲				
flesh only, 150 g	150	40	8					▲				
whole fruit, 300 g	150	40	8					▲				
Grapefruit juice, sweetened, 200 ml	330	80	20					▲				
unsweetened, 200 ml	260	60	10					▲				
Grape juice, 200 ml	530	130	34									
Grapenuts (General Foods), 30 g + 100 ml full-cream milk	730	170	27	△		△			△	△	△	○
+ semi-skimmed milk (2% fat)	680	160	28	△					△	△	△	
Grapes, with skin and pips, 150 g	330	75	20			△						
flesh only, 150 g	390	90	24			△						
Greengages, raw, with stones, 150 g	290	68	17									
without stones, 150 g	300	75	18									
Greengages, stewed with sugar, weighed without stones, 150 g	450	110	30									
with stones, 150 g	480	115	30									

Table 2

Gr-Je

Key △ = ¼ RDA
▲ = ½ RDA
○ = 20+ % fat
● = 40+ % fat

	Kilojoules	Kilocalories	Carbohydrate	Protein	Calcium	Iron	Vitamin A	Vitamin C	Riboflavin	Thiamin	Niacin	Fat
Greengages, stewed without sugar, weighed with stones, 150 g	240	55	15									
without stones, 150 g	255	60	17									
Grouse, roast, weighed with bone, 300 g (150 g edible)	1500	360	0	▲		▲			▲	▲	▲	○
Guavas, canned in syrup, 150 g	400	90	25					▲				
Guava, whole, raw, 150 g	375	90	23					▲				
Gums, fruit, 100 g	750	180	45									
Haddock, fried, 200 g	1400	340	0	▲	△	△					△	●
weighed with bones, 200 g	1300	300	0	▲	△	△					△	●
Haddock, smoked, steamed, 200 g	860	200	0	▲	△	△					△	
weighed with skin and bones, 200 g	550	130	0	△							△	
Haddock, steamed, 200 g	840	200	0	▲	△						△	
weighed with skin and bones 200 g	650	150	0	▲							△	
Haggis, 200 g	2600	600	40	△		▲	▲		△	△		●
Halibut, steamed, weighed with skin and bones, 200 g	800	200	0	▲							△	○
Halva (Greek), 50 g	1300	310	27		△							●
Halwa (Indian), 50 g	800	190	14									○
Ham, canned, 200 g	1000	240	0	▲		△			△	▲	△	●
Ham and pork, chopped, canned, 200 g	2200	520	0	△		△			△	△	▲	●
Hamburger, dieter's (1) ●	1050	250	0	△		△				△	△	●
Hamburger, dieter's (2) ●	1200	290	3	△		△				△	△	●
Hare, stewed, 300 g (150 g meat)	1800	420	0	▲		▲			△		▲	●
Hazelnuts, 30 g	500	120	0									●
Heart, ox, stewed, 200 g	1500	360	0	▲		▲			▲	▲	▲	●
Heart, sheep, roast, 200 g	2000	480	0	▲		▲			▲	▲	▲	●
Herring, fried, 200 g	2000	480	0	▲		△			△		△	●
weighed with bones	1700	400	0	▲		△			△		△	●
Hominy grits (maize), raw, 100 g	1500	360	78									
Honey, 20 g	240	60	15									
Honeycomb, 20 g	240	60	15									
Horseradish, raw, 25 g	60	15	0					▲				
Hot pot, 200 g	1000	240	20	△		△	▲				△	○
Huevos flamencos ●	710	170	7	△		△	▲		△			●
Ice-cream, dairy (milk fat), 150 g	1000	250	37		△				△			○
non-dairy	1000	250	32		△							●
Irish stew, 200 g	1000	240	20									●
Jam, ordinary, 5 ml (level teaspoon)	70	17	4									
"Jam, slimming" (fruit/sugar conserve)	35	9	2									
Jam, traditional types, 20 g	220	50	14									
Jellabi, 50 g	650	155	25									○
Jelly, made with water, 150 g	375	90	23									
with milk	540	135	24		△							

Table 2 (per portion) continued	Kilojoules	Kilocalories	Carbohydrate	Protein	Calcium	Iron	Vitamin A	Vitamin C	Riboflavin	Thiamin	Niacin	Fat
Kedgeree, 200 g	1200	280	20	△		△						●
Kidney, lamb, fried, 200 g	1300	310	0	▲		▲	▲	▲	▲	▲	▲	●
Kidney, ox, stewed, 200 g	1400	350	0	▲		▲	▲	▲	▲	△	▲	●
Kidney, pig, stewed, 200 g	1300	320	0	▲		▲	△	▲	▲	△	▲	●
Kipper, baked, 200 g	1800	420	0	▲	△	△			△		△	●
weighed with bones	900	220	0	△					△		△	●
Ladies, fingers, canned, 150 g	100	25	0		△	▲						
Lager, *see* Beer												
Lamb, breast, roast, 250 g	4200	1000	0	▲		△			△		▲	●
lean only, 250 g	2600	600	0	▲		▲			▲	△	▲	●
Lamb, leg, roast, 250 g	2700	650	0	▲		▲			▲	△	▲	●
lean only	2000	480	0	▲		▲			▲	△	▲	●
Lamb, scrag end and neck, stewed, 200 g	2400	600	0	▲		△			△		△	●
lean only, weighed with fat and bone, 250 g	1300	320	0	▲		△			△		△	●
Lamb, shoulder, roast, 200 g	2600	630	0	▲		△			▲		▲	●
lean only	1600	380	0	▲		△			△	△	▲	●
Lamb chops, weighed with bone, grilled, 250 g	2800	700	0	▲		△			△	△	▲	●
weighed with fat and bone, lean only	1300	300	0	▲		△			△	△	▲	●
Lamb cutlets, grilled, weighed with bone, 250 g	2500	600	0	▲		△			△	△	▲	●
weighed with fat and bone, lean only, 250 g	1000	240	0	△		△			△	△	▲	●
Laverbread, cooked with oatmeal, 150 g	300	75	0			▲		△				
Leeks, raw, 150 g	200	50	0		△			▲				
boiled, 150 g	150	35	0		△			▲				
Lemon, one slice = 10 g	0	0	0					△				
juice, 10 g	0	0	0					△				
Lemonade, bottled or canned, 200 ml	180	40	12									
Lemon curd (made with eggs and lemons), 20 g	240	60	8									
starch-based, 20 g	240	60	15									
Lemon sole, 200 g weighed with skin and bones	1400	340	14	△	△						△	●
Lemon sole, steamed, 200 g	760	180	0	▲							△	
fried, weighed with skin and bones	540	120	0	△							△	
Lentils, cooked, 200 g	850	200	34	△		▲				△		
Lettuce, 150 g	75	15	0				▲	▲				
Lime, one slice = 10 g	0	0	0					△				
juice, 10 g	0	0	0					△				
Liquorice allsorts, 100 g	1300	30	74			▲						
Liver, calf, fried, 200 g	2000	480	0	▲		▲	▲	▲	▲	△	▲	●
Liver, chicken, fried, 200 g	1600	380	0	▲		▲	▲	▲	▲	▲	▲	●
Liver, lamb, fried, 200 g	2000	480	0	▲		▲	▲	▲	▲	△	▲	●

Table 2   Li–Mi

Key
△ = ⅙ RDA
▲ = ½ RDA
○ = 20+ % fat
● = 40+ % fat

	Kilojoules	Kilocalories	Carbohydrate	Protein	Calcium	Iron	Vitamin A	Vitamin C	Riboflavin	Thiamin	Niacin	Fat
Liver, ox, stewed, 200 g	1600	380	0	▲		▲	▲	▲	▲	△	▲	●
Liver, pig, stewed, 200 g	1600	380	0	▲		▲	▲	▲	▲	△	▲	●
Liver, "tarragon wine" *	1550	370	5	▲		▲	▲	▲	▲	△	▲	●
Liver pâté, chicken- *	550	130	0	▲		▲	▲	▲	▲		△	●
Lobster, boiled, 200 g	1000	240	0	▲	△							○
weighed with shell (70% waste), 1000 g	1500	360	0	▲	△	△						○
Loganberries, canned in syrup, 150 g	660	150	40			△		▲				
Loganberries, raw, 150 g	110	25	0			△		▲				
stewed without sugar, 150 g	105	20	0			△		▲				
with sugar, 150 g	350	80	20			△		▲				
Lucozade, 200 ml	580	140	36									
Macaroni, boiled, 200 g	1000	240	50									
Macaroni cheese, 150 g	1100	260	23	△	▲							●
Macaroni cheese *	1550	370	42	△	▲		△		△			●
Mackerel, fried, 200 g	1600	380	0	▲		△			△		▲	●
weighed with bones	1200	280	0	▲					△		▲	●
Mackerel pâté *	500	120	0	△							△	●
Maize (sweetcorn), 200 g	1000	240	46			△	△		△	△		
Maize grits, raw, 100 g	1500	360	78									
Mandarine oranges, see Tangerines												
Mango, raw, 200 g	500	120	30				▲	▲				
canned, 200 g	660	160	40				▲	△				
Margarine, 15 g	460	110	0				△					●
Marmalade, 20 g	220	50	14									
Marrow, boiled, 150 g	45	10	0									
Marrow stuffed with beef *	1700	400	4	▲	▲	△		△	△		△	●
Marrow stuffed with chicken *	1260	300	4	▲	▲			△	△		▲	●
Marzipan, 30 g	550	130	15									●
Masur dahl (from lentils), 200 g	800	190	22		△							○
Mayonnaise, 30 ml	900	210	0									●
Meat, luncheon, canned, 200 g	2600	620	20	△		△					△	●
Meat paste, 50 g	350	85	0									●
Medlars, raw, 200 g	360	80	20									
Melon, Cantaloupe, orange-coloured, flesh only, 200 g	200	50	10				▲	▲				
weighed with skin, 200 g	120	30	7				▲	▲				
Melon, honeydew, yellow, 200 g	180	40	10					▲				
weighed with skin, 200 g	120	30	0					▲				
Melon, water, 200 g	180	40	10					△				
weighed with skin, 200 g	120	30	0									
Meringue (without cream), 30 g	480	110	29									
Milk, goat's, one glass = 200 ml	600	140	9	▲								●
one pint	1700	400	26	△	▲		△	△	▲	△		●
Milk, one glass, whole	540	130	9	▲					△			●
semi-skimmed (2% fat)	450	100	10	▲					△			○

Table 2 (per portion) continued

	Kilojoules	Kilocalories	Carbohydrate	Protein	Calcium	Iron	Vitamin A	Vitamin C	Riboflavin	Thiamin	Niacin	Fat
skimmed	285	66	10	▲					△			
Milk, one pint, whole	1540	370	27	△	▲		△	△	▲	△		●
Millet flour, 100 g	1480	350	75							▲		
Mincemeat, 30 g	360	84	18									
Moules marinières *	1100	260	5	△	▲	▲		▲	△			●
Moussaka, 200 g	1500	360	20	△	△	△			△	△	△	●
Mousse, apricot *	630	150	26	△	▲		△		△			
Mousse, iced melon *	210	50	9	△			△	▲	△			
Mulberries, raw, 200 g	300	70	16			△		▲				
Mushrooms, French *	230	55	0			△						●
Mushrooms, raw, 150 g	75	15	0						△		△	
fried, 200 g	1700	400	0			△						●
Mussels, boiled, weighed with shells (80% waste), 500 g	350	85	0	▲	▲	▲						○
Mussels, boiled without shells, 125 g	350	85	0	▲	▲	▲						○
Mustard and cress, 50 g	25	5	0					▲				
Nectarines, raw, without stones, 200 g	440	100	24				△	△				
weighed with stones, 200 g	400	90	22				△	△				
Noodles, wheat, egg, raw, 100 g	1650	390	72	△		△				△	△	
cooked, 200 g	1000	240	44									
Noodles, wheat, raw, 100 g	1650	390	76	△		△				▲	△	
cooked, 200 g	1000	240	48							△		
Nuts, see named types												
Oatmeal porridge, 200 g, made with water	380	90	16									
Oatmeal porridge, made with 200 ml full-cream milk	735	220	26		▲				△			●
with half-skimmed milk	660	185	25		▲				△			○
with skimmed milk	590	150	24		▲				△			
Oil, vegetable, teaspoon = 5 g	180	45	0									●
Okra, canned, 150 g	100	25	0	△	▲							
Olive oil, teaspoon = 5 g	180	45	0									●
Olives, pickled, flesh only, 50 g	210	50	0									
weighed with stones, 50 g	170	40	0									
Omelet, basic *	840	200	0	△		△	△		△			●
Omelet, beef and asparagus *	1050	250	0	△		△	△		△		△	●
Omelet, cheese and tomato *	1220	290	0	△	▲	△	▲	△	△			●
Omelet, chicken *	1200	290	0	△		△	△		△		△	●
Omelet fines herbes *	840	200	0	△		△	△		△			●
Omelet, lemon soufflé *	880	210	0	△	△	△	△	▲	△			●
Omelet, mushroom *	840	200	0	△		△	△		△			●
Omelet, shrimp *	1100	260	0	△	△	△	△		△			●
Omelet, Spanish *	1520	360	3	△			△	▲	△	△		●
Onions, raw, 150 g	150	36	8					▲				
boiled, 150 g	75	18	5					△				
fried, 100 g	1400	340	10									●

Table 2 Or-Pe

Key
△ = ⅙ RDA
▲ = ½ RDA
○ = 20+ % fat
● = 40+ % fat

	Kilojoules	Kilocalories	Carbohydrate	Protein	Calcium	Iron	Vitamin A	Vitamin C	Riboflavin	Thiamin	Niacin	Fat
spring, raw, 150 g	220	50	14	▲	△	△	▲					
Orange, flesh only, 200 g	340	80	20					▲				
weighed with peel, 200 g	260	60	16					▲				
juice, 200 ml	340	80	20					▲				
Orange juice, canned, unsweetened, 200 ml	340	80	20					▲				
sweetened, 200 ml	380	90	24					▲				
made from concentrate, unsweetened, 200 ml	340	80	20					▲				
Oxtail, stewed, 600 g (150 g edible)	1500	360	0	▲		▲			△		△	●
Oysters, raw, weighed with shell (90% waste), 1000 g	200	50	0	△	▲	▲	△		△			
Oysters, raw, without shells, 100 g	200	50	0	△	▲	▲	△		△			
Pancake, one = 30 g	390	90	11									●
Pancakes, Scotch, two *	380	90	17	△								
Papadums, raw, 100 g	1200	290	46	△	△	▲				△		
Papaya, see Paw paw												
Parsley, raw, 20 g	20	4	0		△	△	▲					
Parsnips, boiled, 150 g	360	90	20					▲				
Partridge, roast, 400 g weighed with bone (160 g edible)	1400	340	0	▲		▲			▲	▲	▲	○
Passion fruit, pulp only, 100 g	150	35	6					△				
whole fruit, 100 g	60	15	0					△				
Pastilles, 100 g	1100	260	62									
Pâté, mackerel *	500	120	0	△							△	●
Paw paw, fresh, 200 g	340	80	20				△	▲				
canned, 200 g	560	140	30				△	▲				
Peaches canned in juice, 200 g	380	90	20				△					
canned in syrup, 200 g	740	180	46				△					
Peaches, dried, stewed without sugar, 200 g	680	160	40			▲	▲				△	
with sugar, 200 g	800	190	46			▲	▲				△	
Peaches, flesh only, 200 g	320	80	18			▲	△					
weighed with stones, 200 g	280	70	16			▲	△					
Peanut butter, 30 g	780	210	4							▲	△	●
Peanuts, fresh, 30 g	720	170	3							▲	△	●
roasted, 30 g	720	170	3							▲	△	●
Pears canned in syrup, 200 g	660	160	40									
canned in water, 200 g	260	60	16									
Pears, cooking, stewed without sugar, 200 g	260	60	16									
with sugar, 200 g	560	130	34									
Pears, weighed whole, 200 g	250	60	15									
Peas, frozen, 150 g	340	80	12			△		▲		△		
boiled, 150 g	260	60	6			△		▲		△		
Peas, garden, canned, 150 g	300	75	10			△		△		△	△	
processed, 150 g	510	120	21			△						

Table 2 Pe-Po
(per portion)
continued

	Kilojoules	Kilocalories	Carbohydrate	Protein	Calcium	Iron	Vitamin A	Vitamin C	Riboflavin	Thiamin	Niacin	Fat
dried, boiled, 150 g	650	150	30			△						
Peas, raw, 150 g	420	100	17			△		▲		△	△	
boiled, 150 g	330	80	12			△		▲	△	△		
Peas, split, boiled, 200 g	1000	240	44	△		△					△	
Peppers, green, raw, 150 g	100	24	0				△	▲				
boiled, 150 g	90	21	0				△	▲				
Pheasant, roast, 400 g (180 g edible)	1600	380	0	▲		▲			△		▲	●
Pickle, piccalilli, 50 g	70	15	0									
sweet, 50 g	300	65	0									
Pie, fruit, individual = 150 g	2400	570	86		△	△						●
pastry top, 150 g	1130	270	42		△				△			●
Pie, lemon meringue, 150 g	2100	500	70				△	△				●
Pigeon, roast, weighed with bone, 500 g (145 g edible)	1400	330	0	▲		▲					▲	●
Pilchards, canned in tomato sauce, 200 g	1000	240	0	▲	▲	▲			△		▲	●
Pineapple, fresh, 200 g	380	90	24					▲				
canned in water, 200 g	380	90	24					▲				
in syrup, 200 g	660	160	40					▲				
Pitta, white (bread), 100 g	1100	260	58	△						△		
Pizza, 150 g	1500	350	38	△	▲							●
Plaice, fried in batter, 200 g	2400	580	30	△	△	△			△	△	△	●
fried in breadcrumbs, 200 g	2000	480	20	▲	△				△	△	△	●
Plaice, steamed, 200 g	800	200	0	▲					△	△	△	
weighed with skin and bones	400	100	0	△								
Plantain, green, raw, 200 g	1000	240	60					▲				
boiled, 200 g	1000	240	60									
ripe, fried, 200 g	2200	540	100					△				○
Plums, dessert, 200 g	320	80	20					△				
weighed with stones, 200 g	300	70	18					△				
Plums, stewed with sugar, 200 g	500	120	30									
weighed with stones, 200 g	460	110	28									
Plums, stewed without sugar, 200 g	180	40	10									
weighed with stones, 200 g	170	38	5									
Polony, 200 g	2400	580	30	△		△				△		●
Pomegranate juice, 200 ml	380	90	24					△				
Popcorn, unpopped, 50 g	750	180	36									
popped, plain, 50 g	800	190	39									
sugar-coated, 50 g	800	190	43									
Pork, leg, roast, 200 g	2400	580	0	▲		△			△	▲	▲	●
lean only, 200 g	1600	360	0	▲		△			△	▲	▲	●
Pork chop, weighed with bone, 250 g grilled	2700	650	0	▲		△			△	▲	▲	●
Pork pie (50% meat), 200 g	3000	720	50	△	△	△				△	△	●
Potato, made from instant powder, 150 g	450	100	24									
Potato crisps, 50 g	1000	240	25			△		△			△	●

Table 2

Key △ = ¼ RDA
▲ = ½ RDA
○ = 20+ % fat
● = 40+ % fat

	Kilojoules	Kilocalories	Carbohydrate	Protein	Calcium	Iron	Vitamin A	Vitamin C	Riboflavin	Thiamin	Niacin	Fat
Potatoes, baked with skin, 150 g	540	130	20					△				
chips, 150 g	1500	360	60					△				○
frozen chips, 150 g	700	170	30					△				○
fried, 150 g	1800	430	45					△				○
mashed (margarine and milk), 150 g	750	180	27					△				○
old, boiled, 150 g	500	120	30					△				
roast, 150 g	1000	240	40					△				○
Potatoes, sweet, boiled, 200 g	760	130	40				▲	▲				
Prawns, boiled, 150 g	700	170	0	▲	▲							
weighed with shell (60% waste), 250 g	700	170	0	▲	▲							
Prunes, stewed with sugar, 200 g	900	220	50					△				
weighed with stones, 200 g	800	200	48					△				
Prunes, stewed without sugar, 200 g	700	160	40					△				
weighed with stones, 200 g	640	150	38					△				
Prune whip *	670	160	28	△	▲				△			
Pudding, black, fried, 200 g	2600	600	30	△		▲						●
Pudding suet, 150 g + 100 g custard	2000	470	63	▲	△	△						●
Puffa Puffa Rice (Kellogg's), 30 g + 100 ml full-cream milk	800	190	30	△	△				△	△	△	
+ semi-skimmed milk (2% fat)	740	175	30	△	△				△	△	△	
Puffed Wheat (Quaker) 30 g + 100 ml full-cream milk	690	160	25	△					△			○
+ semi-skimmed milk (2% fat)	640	150	25	△					△			
Pumpkin, cooked, 150 g	120	30	0				△	△				
Quiche Lorraine, 150 g	2500	600	30	△	▲	△	△		△	△		●
Rabbit, stewed, 400 g (140 g edible)	1600	400	0	▲		△			△		▲	●
Radishes, 50 g	35	8	0					△				
Raisins, 30 g	300	80	20									
Raspberries, canned, 200 g	740	180	46			△		△				
raw, 200 g	200	50	12			△		▲				
stewed with sugar, 200 g	600	140	34			△		▲				
without sugar, 200 g	200	50	12			△		▲				
Raspberry cream *	250	60	16	△	▲			▲	△			
Ready Brek (Lyons), 30 g + 100 ml full-cream milk	770	180	26		△						△	○
+ semi-skimmed milk (2% fat)	720	170	26		△						△	
Rhubarb, canned in syrup, 200 g	400	100	25		△			△				
rhubarb, stewed with sugar, 200 g	400	100	25		△			△				
without sugar, 200 g	50	12	0		△			△				
Ribena, diluted, 200 ml	200	45	12					▲				
Rice flour, 100 g	1530	370	80									
Rice pudding, canned	600	140	23									○
Rice pudding made with full-cream milk	1060	250	39	▲					△			○
with skimmed milk	920	190	41	▲								

119

**Table 2
(per portion)**
continued

	Kilojoules	Kilocalories	Carbohydrate	Protein	Calcium	Iron	Vitamin A	Vitamin C	Riboflavin	Thiamin	Niacin	Fat
Roe, cod, hard, fried, 200 g	1700	400	0	▲		△	△		▲	▲	△	●
herring, soft, fried, 200 g	2000	480	0	▲		△			▲	△	△	●
Rolls, bread, white, crusty 60 g	740	175	34									
soft	770	180	32									
Rolls, bread, wholemeal, crusty	740	175	34									
soft	715	170	29									
Rose-hip syrup, diluted, 200 ml	200	45	12					▲				
Sago pudding, made with full-cream milk, 200 g	1500	360	70		△				△			○
with semi-skimmed milk	1360	300	75		△				△			
Salad, carrot, apple and nut *	630	150	17		△		▲	△		△	△	●
Salad, cheese, orange and watercress *	840	200	10	△	▲		△	▲	△			●
Salad, chicory, orange and watercress *	250	60	8		△		△	▲				
Salad, endive *	340	80	0			△	△	△			△	●
Salad, endive and walnut *	550	130	0					△				●
Salad cream, 30 ml	390	90	5									●
Salad oil, teaspoon = 5 g	180	45	0									●
Salami, 200 g	4000	960	0	▲		△			△	△	▲	●
Salmon, canned, 200 g	1300	310	0	▲	△	△	△		△		▲	●
Salmon, smoked, 100 g	600	140	0	▲					△	△	▲	○
Salmon, steamed, 200 g	1600	380	0	▲					△	△	▲	●
weighed with bones and skin	1300	300	0	△					△		▲	●
Salmon salad *	1500	360	5	▲		△		▲		△	▲	●
Salsify, boiled, 150 g	120	30	0		△	△		△				
Samosas (minced lamb), 100 g	2400	570	9									●
Sardines, canned in oil, drained, 150 g	1350	330	0	▲	▲	▲			△		▲	●
canned in tomato sauce, 150 g	1100	270	0	△	▲	▲			△		▲	●
Sauce, white, low-calorie, 30 g *	170	40	4									●
Sausage, liver 200 g	2600	600	10	△		▲	▲		▲	△	△	●
Sausages, beef, fried, 200 g	2200	520	30	△	△	△					▲	●
Sausages, beef, grilled, 200 g	2200	520	30	△	△	△					▲	●
Sausages, pork, fried, 200 g	2600	600	20	△	△	△			△		△	●
Sausages, pork, grilled 200 g	2600	600	20	△	△	△			△		△	●
Sausage roll, flaky pastry, one = 50 g	1000	240	18									●
Sausage roll, short pastry, one = 50 g	950	230	18									●
Saveloy, 200 g	2000	480	20	△		△					△	○
Scallops, steamed, without shells, 200 g	900	200	0	▲	▲	▲						
Scampi, fried in breadcrumbs, 200 g	2600	600	60	△	△							●
Scones, drop, two *	340	80	12									
Scotch egg, 100 g	1200	280	12	△					△			●
Seakale, boiled, 150 g	45	12	0		△			▲				
Semolina pudding (75 g), made with full-cream milk (200 ml)	1020	250	35		▲				△			○

Table 2   Sh–Su

Key
△ = ⅛ RDA
▲ = ½ RDA
○ = 20+ % fat
● = 40+ % fat

	Kilojoules	Kilocalories	Carbohydrate	Protein	Calcium	Iron	Vitamin A	Vitamin C	Riboflavin	Thiamin	Niacin	Fat
with skimmed milk	870	180	37	▲					△			
Shepherd's pie, 200 g	500	120	20	△	△						△	●
Sherry, dry, 100 ml	480	115	0									
medium, 100 ml	490	116	4									
sweet, 100 ml	570	135	7									
Shredded Wheat (Nabisco), 30 g + 100 ml full-cream milk	690	160	25		△				△	△	△	○
+ semi-skimmed milk (2% fat)	640	150	25		△					△	△	
Shrimp omelet *	1100	260	0	△	△	△	△		△			▲
Shrimps, boiled, 200 g	1000	240	0	▲	▲	△					△	
boiled, weighed with shells (two-thirds waste), 450 g	750	180	0	▲	▲	△					△	
Shrimp surprise *	100	25	0				▲					
Shrimps in tomatoes *	550	130	15	△	△	△	▲				△	○
Skate, fried in batter, 200 g	1700	400	10	▲	▲	▲					△	●
fried in batter, weighed with skin and bones, 200 g	1400	340	8	△	▲	△					△	
Smacks (Kellogg's), 30 g + 100 ml full-cream milk	730	175	31		△	△			△	△	△	
+ semi-skimmed milk (2% fat)	680	160	31		△	△			△	△	△	
Soup, celery *	420	100	14		▲			△	△			
Soup, leek and tomato *	210	50	11		▲			▲				
Soup, watercress and yogurt *	320	75	9		▲			△	△			
Soyabean curd, steamed, 200 g	580	140	0	△	▲	△						●
Special K (Kellogg's), 30 g + 100 ml full-cream milk	720	170	27		△	△			△	△	△	
+ semi-skimmed milk (2% fat)	675	220	31		△	△			△	△	△	
Spinach, boiled, 150 g	200	45	0		▲	▲	▲	▲				
Sponge pudding, 150 g + 100 g custard	2000	470	63	▲	△	△						●
Sprats, fried, 150 g	2700	640	0	▲	▲	▲			△		▲	●
weighed with bones, 150 g	2400	580	0	▲	▲	▲					△	●
Spreads, low-fat, 15 g	225	55	0				△					●
Spring greens, boiled, 150 g	60	15	0		△	△	▲	▲	△			
Squash, raw, 200 g	200	50	10			▲	△					
Steak, stewed with gravy, canned, 200 g	1500	360	2	△		△					△	●
Steak and kidney pie, 200 g	2400	580	30	△		▲	△		▲	▲	△	●
individual pie	2600	620	50	△	△	▲			△	△	△	●
Strawberries, 200 g	200	50	12					▲				
canned in syrup, 200 g	700	160	40					▲				
Sugar, 2 teaspoons, white or brown	250	60	15									
Sugar confectionery, *see specific types*												
Sugar Puffs (Quaker) 30 g + 100 ml full-cream milk	720	170	30		△	△						○
+ semi-skimmed milk (2% fat)	670	155	30		△	△						
Sultanas, 30 g	300	80	20									

Table 2
(per portion)
continued
Su-Ve

	Kilojoules	Kilocalories	Carbohydrate	Protein	Calcium	Iron	Vitamin A	Vitamin C	Riboflavin	Thiamin	Niacin	Fat
Sultana Bran (Kellogg's), 30 g + 100 ml full-cream milk	660	160	25		△	△			△	△	△	○
+ semi-skimmed milk (2% fat)	610	145	25		△	△			△	△	△	
Swede, boiled, 150 g	120	30	0	.				▲				
Sweetbread, lamb, fried, 200 g	2000	480	20	▲		△		▲	△			●
Sweetcorn, boiled, 200 g	1000	240	46			△	△			△	△	
canned, 200 g	600	140	32			△	△					
Sweet potatoes, boiled, 200 g	760	130	40				▲	▲				
Sweets, *see* specific types												
Sweets, boiled, 100 g	1400	330	87									
Syrup, golden, 15 g	190	45	12									
Tangerines, flesh only, 200 g	340	80	20					▲				
weighed with peel, 200 g	260	60	16					▲				
juice, unsweetened, 200 ml	340	80	20					▲				
Tangerine juice, sweetened, 200 ml	380	90	24					▲				
Tapioca pudding (45 g), made with full-cream milk (200 ml)	765	180	23	▲								○
with skimmed milk	525	115	25	▲								
Taramasalata, 100 g	1800	430	4									●
Tofu, canned, fried, 200 g	2600	600	8	▲	▲	▲						●
Tofu, steamed, 200 g	580	140	0	△	▲	△						▲
Tomato juice, canned, 100 ml	70	17	0			△	▲					
Tomatoes, canned, two	50	12	0			△	▲					
Tomatoes, raw, two	60	14	0			△	▲					
fried, two	300	70	0									●
Tongue, canned, 200 g	1800	420	0	△		▲			▲		△	●
Tongue, lamb, stewed, 200 g	2400	580	0	▲		▲		△	▲	△		●
Tongue, ox, pickled, 200 g	2400	580	0	▲		▲			△		△	●
Treacle, 15 g	165	39	10		△	△						
Trifle, 150 g	1000	250	38									○
Tripe, stewed, 200 g	800	200	0	△	▲							●
Trout, steamed, 200 g	1200	280	0	▲		△			△		△	○
weighed with bones, 200 g	800	200	0	▲					△		△	○
Tuna, canned in oil, drained, 200 g	2400	580	0	▲		△			△	△	▲	●
Turkey, roast, 200 g	1400	340	0	▲		△			△		▲	
meat only	1200	280	0	▲		△			△		▲	
dark meat	1200	280	0	▲		△			△		▲	○
light meat	1100	260	0	▲					△		▲	
Turnip, boiled, 150 g	90	20	0		△		△	▲				
Turnip tops, boiled, 150 g	75	18	0		△	▲	▲	▲				
Veal cutlet, fried in egg and breadcrumbs, 200 g	1800	430	0	▲		△			△	△	▲	●
Veal fillet, roast, 200 g	2000	480	0	▲		△			△	△	▲	●
Veal, jellied, canned, 200 g	1000	240	0	▲		△			△		▲	○
Veal pimientos *	420	100	9	△		△	△	▲	△	△	△	○

Table 2   Ve-Zu

Key △ = ⅛ RDA
     ▲ = ½ RDA
     ○ = 20+ % fat
     ● = 40+ % fat

	Kilojoules	Kilocalories	Carbohydrate	Protein	Calcium	Iron	Vitamin A	Vitamin C	Riboflavin	Thiamin	Niacin	Fat
Veal and mushrooms *	1130	270	11	▲	▲	△			▲	△	▲	○
Venison, roast, 150 g	1200	300	0	▲		▲			△		△	○
Vodka, 50 ml	460	110	0									
and mixer, 150 ml	460	110	0									
Walnuts, 30 g	750	180	0									●
Watercress, 100 g	60	14	0		▲	△	▲	▲				
Watercress and yogurt soup *	320	75	9		▲				△	△		
Watermelon, *see* Melon, water												
Weetabix, 30 g + 100 ml full-cream milk	700	170	26		△	△			△	△	△	○
+ semi-skimmed milk	650	155	26		△	△			△	△	△	
Welsh rarebit, 100 g	1500	360	25	△	▲		△					●
Whelks, boiled, weighed with shell (85% waste), 500 g	300	70	0	△		▲						
Whisky, 50 ml	460	110	0									
Whisky and soda, 150 ml	460	110	0									
Whitebait, fried, 200 g	4000	950	0	▲	▲	▲			△		▲	●
Whiting, fried, 200 g	1600	380	15	▲	△				△	△	△	●
weighed with bones	1400	360	12	▲	△				△	△	△	●
Wine, red, 100 ml	280	70	0									
white, dry, 100 ml	280	70	0									
medium, 100 ml	310	75	0									
sweet, 100 ml	400	95	0									
Wine, port, 100 ml	660	160	12									
Winkles, boiled, weighed with shell (80% waste), 500 g	300	70	0	▲								
Yam, boiled, 200 g	1000	240	0									
Yogurt, low-fat, flavoured, 150 g	510	120	21		▲				△			
unflavoured	330	80	9		▲				△			
Yorkshire pudding, 50 g	450	100	13									●
Zucchini, raw, 200 g	200	50	10			▲	△	▲				

Table 3
Dietary fibre
per 100 g

All-Bran (Kellogg's)	26.0
Apple	2.0
Apricots, fresh	2.1
dried, raw	24.0
stewed with sugar	8.5
Asparagus, boiled	1.5
Avocado pear	2.0
Banana	3.4
Beans, butter	5.1
Beans, haricot, cooked	6.1
baked	3.2
Beansprouts, canned	3.0
Beefburger	1.9
Biscuit, chocolate	3.2
creamcracker	6.6
digestive, plain	5.5
chocolate	3.5
ginger nut	2.0
matzo	3.9
oatcake	4.0
sandwich	1.0
semi-sweet	1.0
shortbread	1.0
water biscuit	2.0
Blackberries, raw	7.3
Bread, white	4.5
brown	6.8
wholemeal	8.2
Vitbe	6.4
Hovis	5.7
French stick	5.6
Vienna	4.6
granary	7.1
Scottish batch	4.3
malt	7.0
currant	4.2
rye	4.1
Broccoli tops, boiled	3.3
Brussels sprouts, boiled	3.3
Burger bun	4.4
Bun, currant	2.0
Cabbage	2.7
Carrot	2.3
Cake, fruit	3.7
fancy, iced	2.4
gingerbread	1.4
Madeira	1.4
rock	2.4
sponge	1.0

Table 3
Dietary fibre per 100 g
continued

Cauliflower	1.8
Chapati, fine flour	3.5
brown	10.0
Cherries	1.7
Chicken finger	3.7
Christmas pudding	3.7
Corn Flakes (Kellogg's)	8.4
Crispbread, rye	12.8
Crumpet	2.9
Cucumber	0.4
Currants, black, raw	8.7
dried	6.5
Figs, dried, raw	18.5
stewed with sugar	9.7
Flour, white, bread-making	4.2
brown	7.8
wholemeal	8.1
biscuit	3.8
cake	3.3
household	4.6
chapati, fine	4.6
brown	11.4
rye	5.9
Gooseberries, dessert	3.5
stewed with sugar	2.5
Grapefruit	0.6
Grapes	0.4
Laverbread (coated with oatmeal)	3.1
Leek, boiled	3.9
Lentils, boiled	3.7
Lettuce	1.5
Loganberries, stewed with sugar	5.2
Lychèes, raw	0.5
canned	0.4
Macaroni, cooked	1.7
cheese	0.9
Marrow, boiled	0.6
Melon	1.0
Muesli	7.0
Mushrooms, fried	4.0
Nectarine	2.4
Noodles, plain, cooked	1.3
egg	1.1
Oatmeal	7.5
Onion, raw or boiled	1.3
spring	3.1
Orange	2.0
juice	0
Parsnip, boiled	2.5

Table 3
Dietary fibre per 100 g
continued

Passion fruit, pulp only	15.9
Pastry, shortcrust	2.5
puff	2.6
Peach	1.4
Pear	2.3
Peas, boiled	5.2
Pizza	2.1
Plums, flesh only	3.1
Pork-and-egg pie	1.0
Potato, boiled	1.0
with skin	2.0
Prunes, stewed with sugar	7.7
Puffed Wheat (Quaker)	9.6
Quaker Oats	6.5
Radishes	-1.0
Raisins	6.8
Raspberries, raw	7.4
stewed with sugar	7.0
Rhubarb, stewed with sugar	2.2
Rice, raw	3.0
cooked	1.0
Rice Krispies (Kellogg's)	6.0
Scott's Porage Oats	6.5
Semolina	2.2
Shepherd's pie	3.1
Shredded Wheat (Nabisco)	11.2
Soya, savoury mince	12.9
Spaghetti, cooked	2.0
brown	4.5
canned in tomato sauce	3.0
Spaghetti bolognaise	1.5
Spinach, boiled	6.3
Spring greens	3.8
Strawberries	2.2
Sugar Puffs (Quaker)	5.3
Swede, boiled	2.8
Sweetcorn (corn-on-the-cob), boiled	4.7
Tangerine	1.9
Tart, jam	2.8
Tomato, raw	1.5
Turnip, boiled	2.2
Veal-and-ham pie	2.7
Vesta beef curry	4.4
chicken curry	4.5
chow mein	6.7
Watercress	3.3
Weetabix	9.3
Yam, boiled	3.9